Please return/renew this item
by the last date shown.
Books may also be renewed by
phone or the Internet.

**Hampshire County Council
Library & Information Service**

http://libcat.hants.gov.uk

home health spa

spa

Anna Selby

hamlyn

Recipe notes

Standard level spoon measurements
are used in all recipes.
1 tablespoon = one 15 ml spoon
1 teaspoon = one 5 ml spoon

Both imperial and metric measurements
have been given in all recipes. Use
one set of measurements only and not
a mixture of both.

Ovens should be preheated to the
specified temperature – if using a fan-
assisted oven, follow manufacturer's
instructions for adjusting the time and
the temperature.

Safety note

It is advisable to check with your doctor
before embarking on any exercise or
diet programme. Home Health Spa
should not be considered a
replacement for professional medical
treatment; a physician should be
consulted in all matters relating to
health and particularly in respect of
pregnancy and any symptoms that may
require diagnosis or medical attention.
While the advice and information in
this book is believed to be accurate
and the step-by-step instructions have
been devised to avoid strain, neither
the author nor the publisher can accept
any legal responsibility for any injury or
illness sustained while following the
exercises, treatments and diet plans.

A Pyramid Paperback from Hamlyn

First published in Great Britain in 2000 by Hamlyn,
a division of Octopus Publishing Group Limited
2–4 Heron Quays, London E14 4JP

Copyright © Octopus Publishing Group Ltd 2005

This revised edition published in 2005

ISBN 0 600 61254 6
EAN 9780600612544

A CIP catalogue record for this book is available from the British Library

Printed and bound in China

10 9 8 7 6 5 4 3 2 1

contents

introduction

It is almost a cliché to say that most of us feel we are severely overstretched, trying to balance work, family commitments and a social life. All too often, the only thing most of us do not find time for is ourselves. Therefore the idea of having a relaxing, pampered weekend is bound to appeal to everyone – just a couple of days where you come first.

Many women, and a fair few men, are tempted by the thought of spending a weekend at a health spa. But, distance, time and, of course, money often make such indulgences impossible. That is where *Home Health Spa* comes in. It shows you how to create your own spa at home, without spending a fortune.

The first thing you need to do is create an oasis of time. Choose a weekend that will be just for you, and don't make any other arrangements. Unplug the phone for the whole weekend and switch off the rest of the world. If you have children, ask your partner or their grandparents to take them for the weekend. Alternatively, you can always arrange a reciprocal weekend with another parent, who will then have a free weekend when you take their children.

This does not mean you have to spend the whole time in isolation at home. Each of the three weekends includes at least one special treat, such as a visit to a professional therapist for a massage or an afternoon at the local pool for a swim and a sauna. Apart from this, you should make sure you get out for a breath of fresh air every day. Take a walk, go cycling or do some gardening. You will find that the daily schedules will allow time for these activities.

You may also want to ask a friend to have a weekend spa with you. You can compare notes on how you are feeling as you progress.

However you decide to spend it, the most important thing is to relax and enjoy yourself, and not feel guilty about spending time on what you are doing. There will be very real benefits, even after this short period, and many of the techniques and therapies you make use of on each of the weekend schedules may well become part of your regular routine.

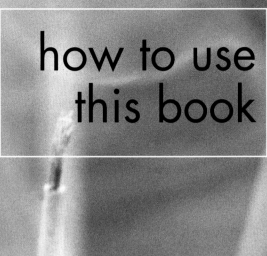

how to use
this book

Home Health Spa is divided into three programmes, each with its own aims and benefits, and each occupying an entire weekend. Therefore the first consideration is what you feel you need and what you want to achieve.

The **Detoxing Weekend** is deeply cleansing and restorative for body and mind. This is the weekend for you if you feel you have a poor diet of rich or junk foods or consume too much alcohol, or if you are continually battling against a polluted smoky atmosphere. It is also very helpful if you have decided to stop smoking; you will feel so purified by the end of the weekend, you may be very reluctant to spoil it all with a cigarette.

The **Relaxing Weekend** is for those who are experiencing prolonged stress. This can manifest itself in any number of ways – anxiety, headaches, digestive problems, depression, skin eruptions or simply feeling unable to cope. By the end of this weekend, you should have brought both the physical and the emotional symptoms of stress under control and be feeling rested and calm.

The **Energizing Weekend** is ideal when you feel under par. You may keep coming down with colds or flu, or feel tired all the time. This weekend boosts the immune system, makes you mentally alert and gives you extra energy.

Whichever programme you decide to try, make sure you read through the whole programme well in advance. Do all of your shopping in advance; you can even cook some of the meals ahead of time and put ready-prepared meals in the freezer to defrost as you need them. There may be other preparations, too. For example, you might want to make a relaxation tape for the relaxing weekend, or book a session with a massage therapist as your special treat. Most importantly, tell everyone you are unavailable that weekend. It is just for you.

Each weekend has a detailed schedule for you to follow. The chapter contents follow the schedule, but where elements are repeated over a weekend, you will need to refer back to an earlier page. Of course, these are your weekends, so feel free to adapt the schedule as you like.

detoxing
weekend

The Weekend

Because this weekend's cleansing diet depends on fresh, preferably organic, fruit and vegetables, buy these on Thursday or Friday so that they are at their best. Look through the recipes you are going to use (see pages 13–15, 21–22, 34–35 and 38–41) and make your shopping list. Keep all fresh produce in the fridge until you need them.

A skin brush and a pot of Moor mud should be available from your local chemist or health shop. And if you are going to a professional for the lymph massage session, don't forget to book an appointment. Also, if you are going to a nearby sauna and steam room on Sunday, remember to book ahead if you need to.

friday

7:00 pm
Evening meal
8:00 pm
Visualization
9:00 pm
Moor mud treatment
10:00 pm
Bed

saturday

8:00 am
Juice
9:00 am
Skin brushing and herb tea or water
9:30 am
Hydrotherapy
10:30 am
Juice
11:00 am
Pilates
12:00 am
Juice
2:00 pm
Herb tea or water
3:00 pm
Manual lymphatic drainage
4:00 pm
Juice

5:00 pm
Herb tea or water
6:00 pm
Visualization
6:30 pm
Juice
8:00 pm
Herb tea or water
10:00 pm
Bed

sunday

8:00 am
Body toning
9:00 am
Breakfast
11:00 am
Swim, sauna and steam
1:00 pm
Lunch
3:00 pm
Hair and skin cleanse
6:00 pm
Evening meal
8:00 pm
Epsom bath
10:00 pm
Bed

friday

7:00 pm Evening meal **8:00 pm** Visualization **9:00 pm** Moor mud treatment **10:00 pm** Bed

friday 7:00 pm **evening meal**

You begin your detox tonight. From now on, throughout the rest of the weekend, you will be eating and drinking only fresh (and, if possible, organic) fruit and vegetables. Because this is such a deeply cleansing diet, you will be throwing off toxins at quite a rate, so you may experience some slightly unpleasant side effects. These can include headaches, skin eruptions, a coated tongue and strange smelling urine. You may also feel tired. None of these is anything to worry about. Take it easy as much as possible and, if you do get a headache, put some lavender oil in a burner or a bowl of hot water and rest to ease it, rather than taking aspirin or paracetamol.

After your supper, therapeutic bath and visualization session, go to bed early and allow the body to start detoxing without any distractions.

Salad supper
You begin the main detox tomorrow with a day of juice fasting. However, tonight you can eat.

Make yourself a big plate of salad, choosing from any of the following recipes. Eat slowly, savouring the fresh flavours. Allow plenty of time for your food to digest by relaxing in a peaceful atmosphere. Part of the aim of this weekend is that your mind should free itself of all negative, stressful thoughts. To achieve this, you need to reverse the all-too-common feeling that we need to be going at full throttle all the time.

You should also start to increase your liquid intake tonight. Drink plenty of bottled or filtered water, or herb tea if you prefer, throughout the evening. This will help to flush out the system and get the detoxing process off to a good start.

salads

Midsummer salad

SERVES 1

½ ripe Ogen melon

1 Little Gem lettuce, shredded

4–5 small strawberries, thinly sliced

2.5 cm (1 inch) piece of cucumber, thinly sliced

1 tablespoon chopped mint

1 tablespoon slivered almonds, to garnish

FRENCH DRESSING

4 tablespoons olive oil

2 tablespoons white wine vinegar

¼ teaspoon French mustard

½ garlic clove, chopped

1 teaspoon clear honey

small strip of lemon rind

few sprigs of herbs

salt and pepper

1 To make the dressing, beat together all the ingredients until they are well blended.

2 Cut the melon into quarters, remove the seeds and the rind. Cut the flesh into cubes, or use a melon scoop to make balls.

3 Place the shredded lettuce on the plate, arrange the melon, strawberries and cucumber on top.

4 Mix the mint into the dressing and pour it over the salad. Serve garnished with the slivered almonds.

Mediterranean salad with grilled vegetables

SERVES 1

1 small fennel bulb

1 red onion

2 courgettes, thinly sliced
lengthways

2 tablespoons extra virgin
olive oil

½ teaspoon finely grated
lemon rind

1 teaspoon chopped
thyme

½ red or yellow pepper,
cored, deseeded and
cut into strips

100 g (3½ oz) cherry
tomatoes, halved

DRESSING

2 tablespoons extra virgin
olive oil

1 tablespoon lemon juice

pinch of sugar (optional)

1 teaspoon chopped
oregano

salt and pepper

1 Cut the fennel bulb and red onion into thick wedges, leaving the root ends intact to prevent the wedges falling apart while they are cooking.

2 Bring a saucepan of water to the boil. Add the fennel and onion. When the water returns to the boil, cook the vegetables for 1 minute. Add the courgette strips to the pan and cook for a further minute.

3 Drain in a colander and refresh under cold running water. Drain the vegetables thoroughly and set aside.

4 Combine the olive oil, lemon rind and thyme in a large bowl. Add the drained vegetables, the pepper strips and the cherry tomatoes. Toss lightly to coat all the vegetables in the oil.

5 Line a grill pan with kitchen foil. Place the vegetable mixture in it, spreading evenly in a single layer. Cook under a preheated hot grill for 15–20 minutes, turning frequently, until the vegetables are tender and patched with brown. Allow the vegetables to cool. Arrange on a plate.

6 To make the dressing, beat together all the ingredients until well blended, pour over the vegetables and serve.

Grilled asparagus salad

SERVES 1

250 g (8 oz) asparagus

2 tablespoons olive oil

25 g (1oz) rocket

25 g (1oz) lamb's lettuce

1 spring onion, finely chopped

2 radishes, thinly sliced

salt and pepper

DRESSING

2 tablespoons extra virgin olive oil

1 tablespoon lemon juice

pinch of sugar (optional)

1 teaspoon chopped oregano

TO GARNISH

roughly chopped herbs, such as tarragon, parsley, chervil or dill

thin strips of lemon rind

1 Trim the asparagus and use a potato peeler to peel about 5 cm (2 inches) off the base of each stalk.

2 Arrange the asparagus spears in a single layer on a baking sheet and brush them with olive oil. Cook under a preheated hot grill for about 7 minutes. Turn the asparagus frequently until the spears are just tender when pierced with the point of a sharp knife and lightly patched with brown.

3 Then, sprinkle with salt and pepper and leave to cool.

4 Arrange the asparagus, rocket and lamb's lettuce on a plate, with the spring onion and radishes.

5 Whisk all the dressing ingredients together in a bowl and then pour it over the vegetables.

6 Garnish with the chopped herbs and lemon rind strips.

friday 8:00 pm **visualization**

Visualization is a form of meditation. Like all meditation, it helps to calm and focus the mind and has many additional benefits: it can improve memory and concentration, relieve stress and any addictive tendencies. If you find yourself craving particular foods or nicotine this weekend, you may well find that visualization will help.

There are several forms that visualization can take, three of which are described below. As its name suggests, visualization is all about seeing an image in your mind's eye. You can achieve this in three ways: by focusing, mental visualization and colour visualization.

Focusing on an object is a good introduction to meditation, as you can remind yourself of what you are doing every time your eye wanders from the object. Mental visualization skips the real object and goes straight to the mental image. Colour visualization appeals to many people, as they find a colour much easier to concentrate on than a more complex image. You may want to try all three methods during the course of the weekend, but keep to one approach each session.

Preparing for visualization

Just as with meditating, when you are in a visualization session, you need to be free from distractions. So unplug the phone and, if there are other people about, ask them to be as quiet as possible and to keep out of the room. However, having someone else with whom to do the visualization exercise can often prove beneficial, adding to the focused atmosphere. Wear loose, comfortable clothing, make sure the room is warm but not stuffy and sit in a position you can hold for up to 20 minutes. You can sit on the floor with your legs crossed or sit in a chair; the most important consideration is to be comfortable and not to have to move during the session.

Before you begin, take a few minutes to settle yourself both physically and mentally. Make sure you are sitting comfortably, and then focus on your mind. There will probably be plenty of thoughts whizzing around in your head, but just watch them, don't get caught up with them. Then place them on one side to deal with when you have finished.

Ideally, your visualization session should last for 20 minutes. If, however, you find this too difficult at first, begin with 10 minutes and try to extend the session a little each time. There will be two sessions a day for the rest of the weekend and the cumulative effect is most beneficial. By the fifth session on Sunday evening you should find your mind is becoming much clearer and calmer. When the session is finished, don't jump up immediately. Remain seated for a few minutes afterwards, breathing slowly and try to retain the tranquillity for the rest of the evening.

Focusing

Choose an object – something small and static, such as a flower, a stone or a lighted candle. Place this in front of you, preferably about 90 cm (36 inches) away and at eye level. Close your eyes and become aware of your body on the floor or chair. Become aware, too, of the noises around you – cars going by, dogs barking, babies crying. Simply observe these sounds and then let them go.

Open your eyes. Look, without blinking, at your chosen object for a minute, or as long as you can. Then close your eyes and look at the image it has left in your mind's eye. When the image fades, open your eyes and look again. Continue in this way, alternating real object with mental image, until the end of the session.

Mental visualization

Close your eyes and picture a place or an object, real or imagined, that you see solely with your mind's eye. Observe this in the greatest detail, focusing on it completely. A place of great tranquillity, such as a deserted beach, has a particularly calming influence.

Colour visualization

Choose a colour and, closing your eyes, try to fill your mind with it to the exclusion of everything else. It may be helpful to start by giving the colour a picture – the blue sea, a snow scene or a field of golden corn. Then gradually try to go in closer so that you can no longer see the outlines of your picture and the colour floods your mind.

friday 9:00 pm **moor mud treatment**

Mud may not be one of the most glamorous forms of treatment in the world, but it is certainly one of the oldest. Mud packs and masks were used by the ancient Egyptians and Romans for healing various ailments as well as being a beauty treatment; they were often given with other spa treatments as part of a cure. Therapeutic mud often originates in areas around mineral springs, and the high mineral content of the mud is regarded as one of the principal reasons for its beneficial effects.

Mud treatments, like spas, are particularly popular throughout Europe. Taking the waters (both drinking them and bathing in them) as well as all-over mud body wraps are frequently seen as important elements of a health regime; for some people, the annual spa 'cure' is very much a part of their lives. People may take cures for specific problems, such as arthritis or psoriasis, or for a more general detoxification of the body.

Although mud treatments are now enjoying something of a revival, people have known of their therapeutic powers for a long period of time. One of the most famous sources of therapeutic mud is the Neydharting Moor, about 60 km (37 miles) from Salzburg in Austria. Archaeological finds on the moor have shown that it was in use from as early as 800BC by the Celts and, later, by the Romans. Sick and injured animals were, and still are, drawn there by its healing powers. Paracelsus, the 15th-century Swiss alchemist and physician, thought that he had discovered the elixir of life in mud. Later visitors included Louis XIV, Napoleon and Josephine, all of whom took the cure.

Known just as 'Moor' or 'Moor-Life', the mud has been investigated and analysed by over 500 scientists, and has been found to be unique. Because the 20,000-year-old glacial valley basin in which it lies was first a lake and then a moor (the waters of which have never drained away), it has retained all of its organic, mineral and trace elements. Other moors have dried out and lost such substances, but clinical analysis has shown that the Moor is uniquely rich in decomposed plant life, with over 1000 plant deposits: flowering herbs, seeds, leaves, flowers, tubers, fruit, roots and grasses. Three hundred of them have recognized medicinal properties, and many of them are extinct or even unique to this one site.

Medical evidence shows that Moor mud's properties are both anti-inflammatory and astringent. This means it is particularly useful for detoxification, in treating skin disorders, such as acne, eczema and psoriasis, and for rheumatism and arthritis. It is used, too, for beauty treatments, to remedy dry hair and to reduce cellulite. Many health shops stock Moor mud treatments and it is also available by mail order.

The Moor drink

The mud comes in a variety of forms, but the ones recommended here are the Moor bath and the Moor drink. Drinking mud does not sound very appetizing and, it has to be admitted, it does actually look like mud, which doesn't help. However, a teaspoonful mixed in a glass of water or fruit juice may colour the liquid but has neither taste nor odour. Take the drink about half an hour before you prepare for the Moor mud bath.

The Moor mud bath

The best time for your bath is immediately before you go to bed. Make sure the bathroom is warm and run a deep bath, pouring in the Moor mud according to the instructions on the container. Mix it in well, or you will end up with muddy globules floating around in the water. Put some warm towels close to the bath to use when you come out.

Lie in the bath for 20–30 minutes. Splash the water on your face, too. You can also rinse it through your hair, if you don't mind having to dry it before you get into bed. Just try to relax in the bath, perhaps with some quiet music in the background. When you are ready to get out, only pat yourself dry – don't rub the towel over your skin. The idea is that you want to leave as much residue from the bath on the surface of your skin as possible. Hop into bed as soon as you are dry.

Moor mud is unique. Scientists have found it contains over 1000 different plant deposits, which give the mud its rich mineral composition.

saturday

8:00 am Juice	**3:00 pm** Manual lymphatic
9:00 am Skin brushing and herbal tea or water	drainage **4:00 pm** Juice
9:30 am Hydrotherapy	**5:00 pm** Herb tea or water
10:30 am Juice	**6:00 pm** Visualization
11:00 am Pilates	**6:30 pm** Juice
12:00 am Juice	**8:00 pm** Herb tea or water
2:00 pm Herb tea or water	**10:00 pm** Bed

Today is the main day of your detoxing, with the juice fast at its centre. Don't be too daunted by a liquid-only day; many people rather enjoy it. Fresh juice has a remarkably cleansing and regenerating effect on the entire system, as juices retain all of the nutrients that can be destroyed during manufacturing processes and during cooking. They are packed with antioxidants to accelerate healing and are low in calories. They are particularly effective at cleansing the gut.

Juices are very easily assimilated by the body and contain all the nutrients present in raw fruit and vegetables, minus most of the fibre. Because it is easier to drink juice than it is to eat huge quantities of raw vegetables or fruit, you may find that you include a larger quantity of fresh, natural nutrients in your diet than usual – which is a good thing.

You cannot make juice with a food processor or liquidizer unless there is a separate juicing attachment. These machines will make a fruit or vegetable purée, while a juicer separates the fibrous pulp from the liquid juice. If you do not have a juicer, you can purchase fresh juice in supermarkets or health food shops. Make sure they do not have any additives.

Preparing fruit and vegetables

Try to use organic fruit or vegetables if you can and choose fruit that is ripe: it will be easier to juice and to digest. Don't buy bruised produce or produce that is obviously past its best. All fruit and vegetables, particularly non-organic, need to be very thoroughly cleaned, as you eat the entire thing. Leave on the tops and outer skins – many nutrients lie just below the surface of the skin. You have to remove peach stones but the smaller pips of apples can go through the juicer.

Home-made juice does not look the same as juice from a carton. It can be rather murky-looking, have a much thicker consistency (sometimes with a froth on top) and have a much more powerful taste. You don't need to strain the juice, even if it does have a froth. Give it a stir and drink it as soon as you have made it. It's best just to make what you need as it loses its nutritional value when it stands, even when kept in the refrigerator.

juices

If you don't have a juicer and just want to buy the juice, adapt the following menu according to what is available. The recipes for the juices can be found on page 22.

- 8:00 am
  The juice of a lemon squeezed into hot water
- 9:00 am
  Herb tea or water
- 10:30 am
  Apple and carrot juice
- 12:00 pm
  Tomato juice
- 2:00 pm
  Herb tea or water
- 4:00 pm
  Raspberry and peach juice
- 5:00 pm
  Herb tea or water
- 6:30 pm
  Apple and carrot juice
- 8:00 pm
  Herb tea or water

Freshly made juices are packed full of vitamins and minerals, taste fantastic and are great for detoxing.

Apple and carrot juice

SERVES 1

Simply delicious, this juice is the best general tonic for cleansing and boosting the immune system. If you choose only one juice, this is the one.

4 carrots

2 green apples

Wash and chop the carrots and apples, if necessary, to fit in the juicer. Juice and drink immediately.

Tomato juice

SERVES 1

This is a vivid, bright red juice. The tomatoes contain betacarotene, which helps to boost the body's immunity to disease, and lycopene, which is a powerful antioxidant that can help prevent cancer.

6 tomatoes

Wash the tomatoes and cut them in half, if necessary, to fit in the juicer. Juice and drink straight away.

Raspberry and peach juice

SERVES 1

This thick, sweet juice is a wonderfully restorative one. It is particularly good if you are overtired or anaemic. If you find it too thick to drink, add an apple or two.

1 small punnet of raspberries

2 peaches

Wash all the fruit and stone the peaches. Juice and drink immediately.

Topping up the liquids

Even though you are having nothing but liquid during the course of the day, juice alone will not be enough. You need to drink about 1.8 litres (3 pints) of extra fluids as well. Plenty of water, filtered or bottled, is most important. It helps to flush out the toxins from your system.

If you want to drink something warm, herbal teas are an excellent way of increasing your fluid intake. They do not contain tannin or caffeine as they are made from pure herbs or, in some cases, spices. You can either make your own with herbs from the garden or the supermarket or buy them ready-made. Whether you use fresh or dried herbs or tea bags, you should let them infuse for at least 5 minutes in boiling water before you drink them.

saturday 9:00 am **skin brushing**

The skin is the largest organ of the body, and the largest area from which toxins are eliminated. There are a number of treatments to stimulate this elimination, of which skin brushing is one. It improves the circulation of blood and lymph, which helps the body to slough off toxins more quickly and efficiently. Skin brushing makes the skin glow by removing the top dull, dead layer. The gentle massaging motion of the bristles also has a beneficial effect on areas of cellulite.

The skin brushing technique is a simple one and you need only a body brush with natural bristles or a loofah. There are various types of body brush, almost all of which are widely available at pharmacies and health or beauty stores.

You will need a brush with a handle – some have detachable handles – so you can reach your back. There are also brushes mounted on long straps, which are ideal for the back and buttocks, and most loofahs are long enough to reach over the shoulders and down the back.

The method
Carry out skin brushing in the bathroom, as you will have your hydrotherapy shower and treatments immediately after. Skin brushing always comes first, as it is always done on dry skin. Make sure the bathroom is warm and there are plenty of towels. Undress and find somewhere comfortable to sit so that you can easily reach your feet and lower legs.

1 Take the brush and begin with the sole of your right foot. Use firm, rhythmic strokes to cover the sole several times. Next, brush the top of your foot, brushing up towards your ankle. Then go on to your lower leg, making sure you cover the whole surface – shin and calf. Always brush in an upwards direction.

2 Stand up and brush the area from your knee to the top of your thigh. Make sure you cover the whole area several times, using long, rhythmic strokes. Brush your buttock area as far as your waist. Now repeat the whole procedure on your left leg, starting again with the sole of your foot.

3 Starting from the top of your buttocks, and always using upwards movements, brush the whole of your back several times all the way up to the shoulder.

4 Next, brush your right arm. Start with the palm of your hand, move on to the back of your hand and then brush from your wrist up to your elbow, always in an upwards direction and ensuring that the whole surface of your skin is brushed. Brush your upper arm, always working from your elbow towards your shoulder, again covering the whole surface of your upper arm. Repeat on your left side, starting again with your hand.

5 Very gently, brush your abdomen. Here, you brush in a circular fashion, always in a clockwise direction. Cover the area several times but with less pressure than on your arms and legs. If it feels uncomfortable, stop.

6 The neck and chest are also very sensitive areas, so, again, brush here very gently. Always work towards your heart. If the bristles are too hard on your neck, don't brush here.

Brushing the whole body in this way will take between 3 and 5 minutes, depending on how many strokes you give to each area. Try to keep a rhythm going and brush for up to 5 minutes. If you do skin brushing on a daily basis, you will find a real improvement in your skin's texture – it tends to become very soft – and it will develop a rosy glow.

Hydrotherapy embraces a far-ranging collection of treatments using water. As with skin brushing, the effect of much hydrotherapy is to jumpstart the system, stimulating the circulation of the blood and the lymph. This is often achieved by extremes of temperature and you quite quickly become accustomed to it. Saunas, steam baths and Epsom baths are all aspects of hydrotherapy, but you begin the morning with a shower.

saturday 9:30 am **hydrotherapy**

Hydrotherapy shower

The bathroom must be warm while you have this shower and there should be plenty of warm towels to hand when you finish. Begin by showering for 2 minutes in warm to hot water. Turn under the shower to make sure your whole body is covered in the water. Now turn the tap to cold and, again, turn your body under the shower so it covers you for 30 seconds. Turn the water back to hot for another 2 minutes, then to cold for a further 30 seconds. Repeat the whole process once more, finishing on cold.

Turning your head so that the cold water pours on to your face is very beneficial for your complexion.

Get out and wrap yourself in warm towels. Pat yourself dry and put on a warm dressing gown. Sit or lie down for at least 10 minutes.

If you find the shower quite tiring, rest until it is time for body toning. However, if you find it stimulating, you might want to try one or two other hydrotherapy treatments. They are very beneficial during detoxification and will often give you a boost if you are feeling tired. If you wish, try one of the following.

Sitz bath

This treatment also works on alternating hot and cold water. Here, you sit in the water. You need two bowls – washing-up bowls or bowls of a similar size.

1 Fill one bowl with very cold water; if you are feeling daring you could even put ice cubes in it. Fill the other with hot water (but test it first, you do not want it scalding hot).

2 You can wear a top to keep your upper body warm, but it should not be a long one that could fall into the water and get wet. Start with your bottom in the hot water and your feet in the cold. This will be quite a shock to the system at first, but after a minute or two, you will start to feel quite comfortable. After 5 minutes, change over bowls so that your bottom is in the cold water and your feet are in the hot. Dry yourself, wrap up in a dressing gown or hop into bed and rest.

Water treading

This involves somewhat less of a shock to the system than the Sitz bath as it involves only the feet. Wrap up to keep as warm as possible, but make sure your clothes do not fall below the knees. Your feet and lower legs should be bare.

Fill the bath with cold water, again making it as cold as possible. Now step into the bath and walk in the water on the spot, lifting your foot out of the water after each step. (Take care that the bath is not slippery. Put a rubber mat on the bottom if it is.) Tread water like this for 1 or 2 minutes. Get out of the bath, dry your feet well and put on a pair of warm socks.

Rest afterwards for at least 10 minutes.

saturday 11:00 am **pilates**

When fasting, even for one day, over-energetic exercise is not appropriate, but a certain amount of gentle exercise will help the detoxification process and also make you feel good. People often assume that while they are fasting they will spend all of their time relaxing. In fact, if you were to lie in bed all day, your system would become sluggish, which is exactly the opposite of what you need while detoxing. Exercise also lifts the spirits, so it helps, too, to overcome feelings of tiredness or lethargy.

The exercises here are based on the Pilates technique, which is a very focused form of exercise. You concentrate on using specific muscle groups correctly to tone, strengthen and elongate and, at the same time, release tension and improve posture. Wear loose, comfortable clothing (cotton is preferable) for exercising and use a room that is warm but not stuffy.

Opening up the upper body

1 Sit on a chair so that your knees are bent at right angles to your thighs when your feet are flat on the floor. Sit with a straight, long back and with your head held high. Focus straight ahead and let your arms hang by your sides. Pull in your stomach muscles (imagine pulling your navel towards your spine) and tense the muscles all around your ribs and waist.

2 Lift your shoulders up as high as you can, then let them drop right down – don't just place them down.

3 Fold your arms loosely in front of you at the height of your breastbone. Your hands should be relaxed, not gripping the arms. Breathe in and, as you breathe out, draw your navel gently towards your spine and start to turn from the waist.

The Pilates method of exercise was developed in the 1920s by the legendary physical trainer Joseph H. Pilates.

4 Turn as far as you can to the side, leading with your elbows and making sure that the turn is from the waist only. Your hips should stay absolutely still.

Turn your head to follow the movement. When you have turned as far as you can, breathe in and return to the centre. Then, repeat on the other side and alternate until you have turned each way 10 times.

Strengthening the abdominals

1 Lie on your back with your knees raised and feet flat on the floor. Your entire spine should be on the floor as well. Make sure your spine is completely straight and that your neck is long, with no tension in your shoulders. Let your arms rest comfortably at your sides.

2 Take a deep breath and, as you breathe out, draw your navel to your spine so that you become aware of the small of your back pressing on the floor.

Squeeze the muscles at the base of your buttocks, not your thighs. Then very slowly start to curl up off the floor, bringing your buttocks and your lower back up in a scooped-out shape. You should have no tension in the shoulders or neck, which stay relaxed on the floor throughout.

Only come up as far as you can. If your abdominal muscles quiver or bulge out, you have come too far. Keeping the movement very slow and focused, repeat up to 10 times.

3 Lie on the floor in the same position as step 1. Put a cushion under your head and shoulders if this feels more comfortable. Place your hands on your thighs.

4 Breathe in and, as you breathe out, press your navel to your spine and slowly start to slide your fingers up your thighs towards your knees. As you do so, your head and shoulders will start to curl up off the floor.

Don't expect to come up too high. It is more important to use the muscles correctly than to come up a long way off the floor. Again, if your abdominal muscles bulge or quiver, you have come too high.

When your fingers have reached as far as they can, place your hands flat on your thighs again, breathe in and slide your hands down, uncurling your back on to the floor. Repeat up to 10 times.

5 Adopt the same starting position as step 1, but this time your right hand supports your head and your left arm rests at your side.

Breathe in and, as you breathe out, press your navel to your spine and slowly reach your left hand towards your feet. This will make your head and left shoulder curl off the floor. Only go as far as you can. Curl back down to the floor and repeat, reaching to the right this time. Build up to 10 repetitions each side.

Arm toners

1 Lie on your back, with your knees lifted and feet flat on the floor, slightly apart. The whole spine should be long and touching the floor, with no tension in the neck or shoulders. Hold a weight of about 1 kg (2 lb) in each hand and place your arms out to the side.

2 Breathe in and, as you breathe out, draw your navel down towards your spine. Breathe out and lift your arms up so that they form a wide circle, as if they reaching around a huge ball. Breathe in and open your arms out to the side, still keeping the curved shape. Breathe out and return, repeating 10 times.

Toning the legs and buttocks

1 Lie on your right side with your back flat against a wall. Stretch your right arm above your head and let your head rest on it; use a cushion if you feel more comfortable. Make sure your left leg makes one long line with your body. Bend your right knee in front of you.

2 Breathe in. As you breathe out, stretch your left leg away from you in a long, low lift, meanwhile keeping the whole of your back flat against the wall. Check with your left hand that your hip doesn't move. Breathe in and lower. Repeat slowly 10 times, and then repeat on your right leg.

3 Now, bend your top leg, keeping your back flat against a wall. Straighten the lower leg so that it is in line with the body.
Breathe in and, as you breathe out, press your navel to your spine and lift the lower leg slowly up and down. Now repeat with the other leg. Build up to doing 10 repetitions on each side.

saturday 3:00 pm **manual lymphatic drainage**

Any type of massage will help you to relax. However, for this weekend, one in particular is of the greatest help in the actual process of detoxification, as well as contributing to a feeling of well being. Known as manual lymphatic drainage, this is a very gentle, rhythmical technique which, by stimulating the lymphatic system, accelerates the process of shedding toxins. Manual lymphatic draining is now widely available. If your local sports centre, gym or pool offers massage, ask if any of the therapists have trained in this type of massage and book an appointment for a treat.

The lymphatic system resembles the circulation system, with the major difference that it does not have a central organ, like the heart in the circulatory system, to keep the lymph fluid moving. Rather, the lymph moves as a result of the muscles contracting and relaxing, hence the beneficial effects of exercise on the lymphatic system. Keeping the lymph moving is vital because it plays such a central part in the health of the immune system. Essentially, it is a waste disposal system. It gets rid of toxins and dead cells, particles of pollution and antibiotics. So, by stimulating the lymphatic system, detoxification becomes more efficient, too.

Manual lymph drainage, by accelerating the workings of the lymphatic system, reduces many of the symptoms that are caused when it is overstretched. These include bloating, cellulite and premenstrual tension. It is also an extremely relaxing therapy, and the very gentle strokes that are used make it ideal during fasting when you may be feeling particularly sensitive.

If you are unable to find a manual lymphatic drainage therapist, there are some very effective ways of stimulating the lymphatic system. One is rebounding – jumping on a mini-trampoline – for about 10–15 minutes. Alternatively, a brisk walk is an excellent way of stimulating the lymph. The more pleasant the surroundings, the better the walk. Go to the country, the seaside or a park. Wear loose, comfortable clothes and low-heeled shoes. Walk at a brisk pace, but don't jog. Enjoy the surroundings, breathe deeply and walk for at least an hour.

Following this, spend the rest of the day relaxing. Between resting and juices, you should fit in another visualization session for 20 minutes. Before bed, you can, if you wish, have a relaxing bath to put you in the mood for a restful night's sleep. Try either the Moor mud bath from Friday night (see pages 18–19) or the Epsom bath (see page 47). Alternatively, if you would like something a little more sensual, you could try the aromatherapy bath from the Relaxing Weekend (see pages 56–57). Whatever you decide, aim to be in bed by about 10 pm.

sunday

8:00 am	**3:00 pm**
Body toning	Hair and skin cleanse
9:00 am	**6:00 pm**
Breakfast	Evening meal
11:00 am	**8:00 pm**
Swim, sauna and steam	Epsom bath
1:00 pm	**10:00 pm**
Lunch	Bed

Today you will be eating solid food, but the detoxification process will continue as you are eating only raw food, and some very lightly cooked fruit and vegetables. Try to drink just as much water as yesterday and include herbal teas whenever you like. The greater the quantity of these fluids you drink, the quicker the toxins will be flushed through the system.

After another session of body toning, as yesterday, it's time for a fruity breakfast. You can just mix up whatever appeals to you and looks good when you go shopping. See the breakfast selection opposite for a few ideas. Try to buy organic produce whenever possible and make sure it is ripe and therefore at its most delicious. You can also have fruit juice and a herb tea to drink.

breakfasts

Tropical temptation

SERVES 1

1 mango

½ pineapple, or 1 small pineapple

6 strawberries

4 tablespoons pineapple juice

honey, to taste (optional)

1 Peel the mango and pineapple and cut them into cubes, discarding the pineapple core. Hull the strawberries.

2 Pour the pineapple juice over the fruit and leave to soak for 30 minutes. If the fruit is ripe this should sweeten it enough. However, if it is too tart for your taste, add a little honey.

Stuffed figs

SERVES 1

3 ripe figs

1 tablespoon ground almonds

25 g (1 oz) raspberries

honey, to taste (optional)

1 Remove the stalks from the figs, make a criss-cross cut at the stalk end and carefully ease them open.

2 Mix the almonds and raspberries together and spoon them into the open figs, adding a little honey to sweeten if you wish.

Kiwi fruit and ginger cup

SERVES 1

½ Ogen melon, deseeded

1 kiwi fruit, thinly sliced

250 g (8 oz) white grapes, halved

½ teaspoon grated root ginger

4 tablespoons apple juice

1 Cut the melon piece in half, remove the seeds and the rind. Cut the flesh into cubes, or use a melon scoop to make balls.

2 Place the melon, kiwi fruit and grapes in a bowl. Scatter with the ginger and then pour the juice over the fruit. Serve immediately.

sunday 11:00 am **swim, sauna and steam**

Sunday's hydrotherapy takes you out to your local gym or swimming pool. Ideally, you should look for a leisure centre that has a swimming pool, sauna and steam room. You can, however, improvize. The other alternative, if you don't have a local pool, or you simply don't feel like going out, is to repeat yesterday's hydrotherapy at home.

In the pool

Swimming is the ideal exercise for a detoxing weekend. You use most of the muscle groups in your body if you vary your strokes, but your muscles and joints are supported by the water, so you are not going to injure yourself, as you might do in an overly energetic aerobics class. It is not necessary to swim at a furious pace or for a long period of time and, if you alternate swimming with the other hydrotherapy methods, your mind and body will feel completely relaxed afterwards.

You can also do some exercises in the water that are particularly beneficial if your joints are stiff. They also help to improve muscle tone, as you are working against the resistance of the water. Warm up first with a couple of lengths and, if you start to feel cold, have another swim.

Exercises for legs and hips

1 Stand so that your side is next to the edge of the pool and hold on to the handrail. With a straight back, lift your outside leg and swing it back and forth as far as you can. Perform 10 repetitions and then change legs.

2 Walk on the spot, feeling your feet go down through your toes to your heels every time you replace them on the floor of the pool. Gradually make the steps bigger, with your knees coming higher each time. If you can, after 2 minutes, turn this into a run. Continue running for 2 minutes.

Exercises for the upper body

1 Standing away from the edge of the pool, with your feet apart and your hands on your hips.

2 Turn as far as you can to the right and then to the left. Repeat 10 times, alternating from side to side.

3 With your shoulders under the water (you can kneel for this if the water is very shallow) take your arms out to your sides so that they are just under the water.

4 With a slight curve from shoulder to your wrist, slowly bring your hands together against the resistance of the water. When your forearms meet, there should be a large circle of water between your arms – enough to encompass a beach ball. Slowly repeat the exercise 10 times.

Sauna and steam

Alternating saunas and steam baths with a cold shower or a swim in the pool works on the hydrotherapy principle of stimulating the circulation of blood and lymph by changing the temperature. Of course, you sweat off waste in the sauna or steam bath, too, which aids detoxification further.

Many sports centres now have saunas and steam baths. If your local centre has ones next door to each other, this is ideal. But, do remember that a very light diet combined with sudden changes of temperature may make you a little light-headed, so walk from one to the other slowly. If you want to have a fairly lengthy swim, do this first.

If for some reason you can only do this part of the detox programme in the afternoon, make sure at least two hours have passed since your last meal. Take off all your jewellery and, for maximum benefit, wear as little as possible.

Alternate 5–10 minutes of heat with 1–2 lengths of the pool, and repeat this a few times. If you don't have a pool, have a cool to cold shower and rest for a few minutes before returning to the heat treatment. Drink plenty of water throughout. Dry yourself gently, then rest, lying down, before you get dressed and go home.

salads

Lunch and evening meal

Sunday's lunch and evening meal are salads.
If you can, eat at least one salad meal a day for
the week following your detox and drink plenty
of water; this will allow the cleansing process to
continue. All of the recipes here are for four small
or two large servings. You can, of course, have
two smaller salads at the same meal.

Continental mixed salad

SERVES 2 OR 4

1 red oakleaf lettuce,
   separated into leaves

½ head of frisé lettuce,
   separated into leaves

50 g (2oz) rocket

50 g (2oz) lamb's lettuce

handful of herbs, such as
   dill, chives and basil

1 red onion, thinly sliced

1 large, ripe avocado

1 tablespoon lemon juice

25g 1oz pine nuts,
   toasted

handful nasturtium flowers
   (optional)

salt and pepper

1 quantity of Tarragon
   dressing (see Jersey
   Royal and celery salad,
   opposite)

1 Tear the oakleaf
leaves and the frisé into
bite-size pieces. Put
them in a large salad
bowl with the rocket,
lamb's lettuce, herbs
and red onion.

2 Peel, halve and stone
the avocado. Roughly
chop the flesh and
place in a small bowl
with the lemon juice.
Toss gently.

3 Just before serving,
add the avocado, pine
nuts and flowers to the
salad and season with
salt and pepper to
taste. Spoon the
tarragon dressing over
the salad, toss gently
and serve straight away.

Jersey Royal and celery salad

SERVES 2 OR 4

500 g (1 lb) small Jersey Royal potatoes, scrubbed

6 celery sticks, with leaves

75 g (3 oz) black olives

3 tablespoons capers, rinsed and drained

few sprigs of parsley, roughly chopped

salt

pepper

TARRAGON DRESSING

2 tablespoons tarragon vinegar

1 teaspoon finely grated lemon rind

¼ teaspoon Dijon mustard

5 tablespoons olive oil

salt and pepper

1 Bring a saucepan of water to the boil. Add the potatoes and boil for about 12 minutes until just tender. Drain the potatoes and leave to cool.

2 Slice the celery sticks diagonally and roughly chop any leaves. Place in a bowl with the olives, capers and parsley. Add the cooked potatoes and season with salt and pepper to taste.

3 To make the dressing, beat together all the ingredients until well blended. Pour the dressing over the salad, toss well and serve.

Lamb's lettuce with mango and mint

SERVES 2 OR 4

1 large mango

1 tablespoon chopped mint

1 tablespoon lime juice

250 g (8 oz) lamb's lettuce

125 g (4 oz) roasted cashew nuts

handful of nasturtium leaves and flowers, to garnish (optional)

YOGURT DRESSING

150 ml (¼ pint) natural yogurt

1 tablespoon lemon juice

1 teaspoon clear honey

½ teaspoon Dijon mustard

salt and pepper

1 Peel and stone the mango and then chop it into bite-size pieces. Place them in a bowl with the mint and lime juice and mix well.

2 Place the lamb's lettuce in a salad bowl. Add the prepared mango and throw in the cashew nuts.

3 To make the dressing, beat together all the ingredients until well blended. Drizzle the dressing over the salad and toss lightly. Garnish with nasturtium leaves and flowers.

French bean and apricot salad

SERVES 2 OR 4

500 g (1 lb) French beans, topped and tailed

6 ripe apricots, halved, stoned and sliced

few sprigs of parsley, roughly torn

1 tablespoon chopped tarragon

1 quantity Tarragon dressing (see Jersey Royal and celery salad, page 39)

salt and pepper

25 g (1 oz) almond flakes, toasted, to garnish

1 Cook the French beans for 2–3 minutes in a saucepan of boiling water. Drain well and place in a salad bowl.

2 Add the sliced apricots to the beans, then add the parsley and tarragon. Season with salt and pepper.

3 Pour the dressing over the salad and toss lightly. Garnish the salad with the almond flakes and serve.

Cottage garden salad with strawberries

SERVES 2 OR 4

250 g (8 oz) mixed salad leaves, such as dandelion, rocket, red oakleaf, radicchio and lamb's lettuce

handful of herbs, such as fennel, chives, dill and mint

250 g (8 oz) small strawberries

1 quantity Tarragon dressing (see Jersey Royal and celery salad, page 39)

salt and pepper

1 Tear the lettuce leaves into pieces and place them in a salad bowl. Scatter the herbs over the lettuce.

2 Halve the strawberries and add them to the salad with a little salt and pepper.

3 Spoon the dressing over the salad and toss lightly.

Green salad with walnuts

SERVES 2 OR 4

large bowl of mixed salad leaves, such as rocket, chicory and spinach

½ mild onion, chopped

50 g (2 oz) walnut pieces

1 quantity Tarragon dressing (see Jersey Royal and celery salad, page 39), substituting walnut oil for the olive oil

1 Tear the salad leaves roughly and toss them into a serving bowl with the onion.

2 Lightly toast the walnuts in a dry pan. Chop them and leave to cool.

3 To make the dressing, beat together all the ingredients until well blended.

4 Add the walnuts to the salad and pour the dressing over the top. Toss lightly to mix.

Grilled pepper salad

SERVES 2 OR 4

2 red peppers

2 yellow peppers

2 green peppers

2 garlic cloves, chopped

1 tablespoon chopped parsley

2 sprigs of basil, shredded

5 tablespoons extra virgin olive oil

2 teaspoons balsamic vinegar

salt and pepper

basil leaves, to garnish

1 Preheat the grill to hot. Place the whole peppers on the grill pan and cook, turning occasionally, until the skins are blistered and blackened all over. This will take about 20 minutes. Place the peppers in a paper or polythene bag and secure the top. Leave to cool.

2 When cool enough to handle, hold the peppers over a bowl to catch the juices and remove and discard the charred, papery skins. Remove and discard the core and seeds.

3 Cut the pepper flesh into long thin strips and arrange them in a shallow serving dish. Sprinkle the chopped garlic, parsley and basil over the peppers. Season with salt and pepper.

4 Drizzle the oil and balsamic vinegar over the salad and serve, garnished with torn basil leaves.

Walnuts contain vital omega-3 fatty acids, which can lower cholesterol and improve blood flow.

sunday 3:00 pm **hair and skin cleanse**

The afternoon treatment is a relaxing, deep cleanse for the hair and skin. It helps eliminate toxins, many of which are lost through the skin during the detoxification process. Keep drinking as much water as you can to speed up the process of flushing the toxins out of your body.

The hair treatment

Apply the hair treatment before you cleanse your face. It contains oily substances, so you will probably want to wash your hair once you have finished. But, if you prefer you could leave it on all night and wash it off when you shower tomorrow morning. Choose the treatment according to your hair type, massage it in well, then wrap a towel around your head for the rest of the session. The treatment oils for greasy and dry and damaged hair appear on page 88.

A hair growth stimulant can be beneficial if your hair seems very thin or if you have lost hair because of childbirth, stress or as a reaction to illness or drugs. To make up the mixture, put:

- 10 drops of rosemary oil
- 10 drops of lavender oil
- 5 drops of sandalwood oil

in 50 ml (2 oz) of carrier oil and massage it well into your scalp.

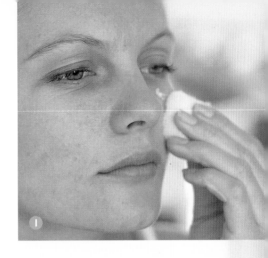

The facial cleanse

You can choose homemade or over-the-counter products for this deep cleansing facial, or a mixture of the two. Follow each stage carefully according to your skin type.

1 Cleanse your face and neck thoroughly to remove all traces of make-up and dirt and pollution from the atmosphere. Either use a cleanser that is applied with water or a cleansing lotion applied with cotton wool. Do not use soap. If you use a cleanser that is applied with water, take a face buff (an object that is like a loofah for the face) and go all over your face using small circular movements to give your skin a mini-exfoliation.

2 Whichever cleansing method you have used, splash some cold water on to your face and neck about 20 times. Then, pat dry.

sunday 3:00 pm **hair and skin cleanse**

3 Exfoliating requires a grainy cleanser that penetrates deeper into the skin and removes all the dry, dead cells on the surface.

There is a wide range of proprietary brand exfoliators, available as gels, liquids, creams and pastes. Choose one that goes on easily so that you don't end up dragging the skin. Alternatively, make your own by mixing together a teaspoonful each of live yogurt, crushed rolled oats and honey. Use small circular movements to cover your whole face and neck, and rinse off with warm water, splashing 20 times. Pat dry.

Apply a mask to your face and neck, but not to your eye area. This will cleanse your face further, drawing out impurities and closing the pores. There are a vast number of over-the-counter masks available and you can choose one according to your skin type. If you prefer, make your own from natural ingredients (see page 88).

4 Apply a chamomile eye compress (see page 89) and lie down and relax.

5 Rinse off the mask completely and spray with the gentle facial toner (see page 88). Apply a moisturizer (again, you can make your own aromatherapy version, try the essential oil skin conditioners on page 88) or simply spread a thin layer of petroleum jelly over your face and neck.

6 Now, simply relax until supper time.

Chamomile has many uses. The Pharaohs of Egypt worshipped it above all others due to its healing qualities.

sunday 8:00 pm **epsom bath**

An Epsom salts bath probably does not sound like a very glamorous end to your weekend. However, it is one of the most cleansing and relaxing late-night treatments imaginable. This is because the magnesium in the Epsom salts warms and soothes the body, so the joints and muscles relax. At the same time, you can expect to get very hot indeed – your body temperature will rise and you will release extra toxins in your sweat.

Epsom salts are available at some pharmacies and health food stores. If you have difficulty finding them, you can substitute herbs and spices; ginger, sage and cayenne pepper have a similar effect in terms of raising the body's temperature.

Caution: Do not use Epsom salts if you have eczema, psoriasis or broken skin. Try the soothing aromatherapy bath instead (see page 56).

The bathroom should be warm and you should have plenty of towels to hand. The salts usually come in 2 kg (4 lb) packs, and you put the whole contents of the pack into the bath. It takes quite a lot of stirring to mix the salts into the water, but do make sure the entire contents of the container have dissolved before you step in and relax.

Soak yourself in the bath for at least 5 minutes. You will start to sweat copiously. However, don't worry, this is completely normal and is part of the process that detoxifies and relaxes your body.

Use a loofah or bath mitt and, beginning with your feet, thoroughly massage with circular movements. Don't try to go too fast or you may become overheated. Work your way up your legs, massaging as you go, then kneel up to work on your buttocks and your abdomen (go gently on the latter). Sit down and work gently over the lower half of your chest, avoiding your breasts, and working over as much as you can of your back.

Lie back and relax for another 5 minutes, if you can. If you find you are becoming too hot, step out of the bath immediately. Wrap yourself in towels and pat your body dry very gently. Do not rub your skin. When you are dry, get into bed and prepare for a long, restful night.

relaxing
weekend

A certain amount of short-term stress is not such a bad thing; as a challenge, it can actually motivate us to achieve a goal. However, in the long term stress can cause all manner of physical and emotional ailments, from migraine and depression to eczema and irritable bowel syndrome.

One of the side effects of stress, and also one of its causes, is lack of time for yourself. You are so busy coping, you forget, or are unable, to relax. The point of this weekend is to reverse this trend. Not only will you give yourself time and several pampering treats, but you will also learn a number of techniques that help to combat stress. Ideally, you should incorporate these into your daily life.

The Weekend

Look through the recipes for the weekend (see pages 52–55, 66–67 and 72–75) and make a list of the food and drink you need to buy in advance. It is a good idea to prepare as much as you can beforehand so you have as few chores as possible during the weekend itself. All of the soups, for example, can be made in advance and frozen until you are ready to use them. You can make your own relaxation tape the week before as well (see pages 68–71). If you decide to go out for a professional massage on Saturday, make sure you book your appointment well in advance.

friday

7:00 pm
Meditation

8:00 pm
Evening meal

9:00 pm
Aromatherapy bath

10:00 pm
Self-massage for sleep

saturday

8:00 am
Yoga

9:00 am
Breakfast

10:00 am
Relaxation and meditation

12:00 am
Lunch

2:00 pm
Massage

4:00 pm
Facial massage

6:00 pm
Evening meal

8:00 pm
Breathing techniques and meditation

10:00 pm
Bed

sunday

8:00 am
Yoga, relaxation and meditation

9:00 am
Breakfast

11:00 am
Acupressure

1:00 pm
Lunch

3:00 pm
Aromatherapy facial

4:00 pm
Meditation

6:00 pm
Evening meal

8:00 pm
Aromatherapy bath

10:00 pm
Bed

7:00 pm
Meditation
8:00 pm
Evening meal
9:00 pm
Aromatherapy bath
10:00 pm
Self-massage for sleep

friday 7:00 pm **meditation**

There are numerous relaxation techniques that can overcome the immediate stresses and strains of contemporary life. However, a period of prolonged stress is another matter; it can manifest itself as high blood pressure, raised cholesterol levels, anxiety, depression and insomnia, among others. To overcome stress-related problems, a quite different form of deep relaxation is needed to disperse severe stress from your body and mind.

Regular meditation has emerged as the most effective way of achieving deep relaxation. A considerable body of scientific research, focusing mainly on the most dramatic and measurable manifestations of stress, such as heart disease and its consequences, has shown that meditation results in substantial reductions in both blood pressure and levels of cholesterol in the blood.

Other clinical tests have shown that the risk of much of the physical and the mental deterioration associated with ageing is reduced considerably in those people who practise regular meditation. Meditation is not, however, merely a preventative medicine; it has many other benefits including:

- physical relaxation

- improved concentration

- increased tranquillity and ability to deal with stress

- improved awareness

- improved creativity and memory.

Preparing for meditation
Meditation is not just day-dreaming or relaxation. Primarily, it is a discipline for training your mind to a point of both deep concentration and relaxation.

During this weekend, you can hope only to achieve an idea of what meditation is like. The first session may seem a little strange, but if you get into a regular rhythm of meditation during the course of these three days, you may well find that its benefits make it something you want to continue.

The main thing to remember when learning to meditate is that the intrusion of thoughts is inevitable. Do not try too hard; you are not supposed to be forcing your mind to concentrate on a particular image. In fact, you are trying to release yourself from conscious thought. When any thought enters your mind, observe its presence gently, make no judgement about the thought itself and, above all, do not become irritated with yourself for having it. Recognize the thought, let it go and draw your focus back to your breath or the word or image on which you are meditating.

You need to be comfortable but alert to meditate; so choose session times carefully so that you're not feeling sleepy. You should also avoid being disturbed. Take the phone off the hook, find a quiet spot, wear loose, comfortable clothing and take off your shoes. You can sit in a straight-backed chair or cross-legged on the floor, whichever you prefer. The important thing is to sit with a straight back and remain still for up to 20 minutes.

Before you begin, take some slow, deep breaths and try to let go of any areas of tension. Scan your mind for immediate thoughts and worries, then leave them on one side so your mind is clear.

Meditation techniques

There are various meditation techniques you can use. Two alternatives are suggested below. Over the course of the weekend, you may want to try both to see if one seems more suitable than the other. However, normally you would give each one 10 days before you decide whether to try the alternative. When you have found a method you like, you should practise it regularly. Try to practise each session at the same time in the same place. When you become more adept, you will be able to meditate at any time in any place.

The breath

Close your eyes and be aware of your breathing. Count each breath, breathing fairly deeply, so that you feel your abdomen rise and fall. Inhale on one, exhale on two, inhale on three, and so on. Your breathing should be even and regular, and you can focus the counting on either the sensation of the air entering through your nose or the rise and fall of your abdomen. If you lose count – and you will – start again at once.

The mantra

This is the silent repetition of a word. It can be a word that has a special significance for you, such as 'peace', or one that has a resonant sound; the best known of these is the word 'om', pronounced 'aum', and pronounced on a slow exhalation of breath. Your aim is to reach a stage where the sound and its resonance fill your mind.

After the allotted time, allow the focus of your meditation to fade away gently and bring your mind back to the present. Take some long, deep breaths and become aware of your body and its sensations, gradually becoming aware, too, of your surroundings and the noises around you. Finally, open your eyes, but remain still for a few more minutes.

You can establish your meditation routine during the course of the weekend – in the morning and in the evening – for the future. It will be particularly beneficial if you meditate after gentle exercise, but avoid practising for at least an hour after a meal. If you find your sessions immediately beneficial, you can add an extra one during the course of the day.

Lunch and evening meals

There are several techniques and treatments that
will aid relaxation of body and mind, and diet has
an important part to play in this. While weight loss
is not the purpose of this weekend, if your body is
working overtime to digest rich food, it is going to
be more difficult to slow down generally. Therefore,
the aim of your diet for the weekend is that it should
be light, nutritious and easy to digest. Your evening
meal each night is a nourishing soup and the main
meal of the day is eaten at lunchtime, when the
body's digestive system is working most efficiently.
If you don't think one bowl of soup will be enough
for you, you can have a second serving, or eat a
slice of wholemeal bread with it.

If you want a restful night's sleep, you should eat
neither too much nor too late in the evening. Don't
be tempted to drink alcohol; although it makes you
feel sleepy initially, it is a stimulant and may well
break your sleep in the middle of the night. Tea and
coffee are also stimulants, so avoid these as well.
Instead, drink plenty of bottled or filtered water
throughout the evening.

Try to eat no later than 8 pm and eat slowly,
concentrating on your food while you eat – don't
watch television or listen to the radio at dinnertime.
This will give your body the chance to slow down.

You may want to make your soup before you
have the meditation session on Friday, so you can
eat it afterwards. You can prepare all the soup for
the weekend in advance, so all you have to do is
get it out of the refrigerator as you need it. All of the
recipes here serve four.

soups

Vegetable stock

Most of the recipes here
call for vegetable stock.
You can buy bouillon
powder or vegetable
stock cubes, but making
your own is simple.

SERVES 4

3 potatoes, chopped

1 onion, chopped

2 leeks, chopped

2 celery sticks, chopped

2 carrots, chopped

1 head of Florence fennel,
chopped

handful of herbs such as
parsley, thyme or bay

1.5 litres (2½ pints) water

salt and pepper

1 Place the vegetables
and herbs in a
saucepan with the
water. Season to taste.
Bring to the boil and
simmer for about
1½ hours, skimming the
surface regularly.

2 Strain the stock
through a sieve and
store in the refrigerator
until required.

Jerusalem artichoke soup

Jerusalem artichokes have a delicious, nutty flavour and make a particularly good soup, ideal for a cold winter's night. Garnish with lemon croûtons.

SERVES 4

500 g (1 lb) Jerusalem artichokes, chopped

3 tablespoons lemon juice

1 tablespoon sunflower oil

900 ml (1½ pints) vegetable stock (see opposite)

1 teaspoon dried dill

½ teaspoon sugar

salt and pepper

LEMON CROÛTONS

4 slices bread, crusts removed

1 tablespoon lemon juice

1 Sprinkle the lemon juice over the artichokes, then heat the oil in a saucepan and add the artichokes, stirring well. Cover and heat gently for 1–2 minutes. Pour in the stock and bring to the boil, then cover and simmer for about 30 minutes.

2 Purée the artichokes and stock in a food processor or blender with the dill and sugar, then push through a sieve and return to a clean pan. Reheat, seasoning with salt and pepper to taste.

3 To make the lemon croûtons, brush both sides of the bread with lemon juice and toast until lightly coloured on both sides. Cut into cubes. Serve the soup warm with the croûtons.

Curried parsnip soup

This is another substantial soup that is particularly good for clearing any respiratory congestion. The sweet taste of the parsnips blends well with the warming effect of the curry. If you prefer a hotter flavour, add more curry powder.

SERVES 4

375 g (12 oz) parsnips, scraped and chopped

1 onion, chopped

600 ml (1 pint) vegetable stock (see opposite)

1 teaspoon mild curry powder

1 tablespoon natural yogurt

salt and pepper

coriander leaves, chopped, to garnish

1 Place the parsnips and onion in a large saucepan with the vegetable stock and season with salt and pepper. Bring to the boil, cover and simmer for 20 minutes or until the parsnips are tender.

2 Remove from the heat and allow to cool slightly, then purée in a blender or food processor, or press through a fine sieve. Stir in the curry powder.

3 Return the soup to a clean pan and reheat. Stir in the yogurt and serve garnished with chopped coriander and parsnip crisps.

Red lentil soup

This satisfying soup is a good choice if you are used to eating a large evening meal.

SERVES 4

250 g (8 oz) split red lentils

1 leek, sliced

2 large carrots, sliced

1 celery stick, chopped

1 garlic clove, crushed

1 bay leaf

1.2 litres (2 pints) vegetable stock (see page 52)

½ teaspoon cayenne pepper

pepper

TO GARNISH

natural live yogurt

finely snipped chives

1 Place all the soup ingredients in a large saucepan, bring to the boil, cover and then simmer for 20–25 minutes or until the lentils and all the vegetables are tender.

2 Allow the soup to cool slightly, remove the bay leaf and purée the soup in a food processor or blender until it is smooth.

3 Reheat the soup, season with pepper to taste and serve warm. Garnish with a swirl of natural yogurt and the snipped chives.

Chilled celery soup

If the weather is warm, you might like to sample this chilled soup. Flavoursome and light, the cumin gives it a hint of richness.

SERVES 4

250 g (8 oz) celery

1.2 litres (2 pints) vegetable stock (see page 52)

1 onion, chopped

250 g (8 oz) potatoes with skins left on, chopped

1 teaspoon ground cumin

3 tablespoons natural yogurt

salt

finely chopped celery leaves, to garnish

1 Thinly slice enough celery to fill two tablespoons. Set this amount aside and grate the remaining celery in a food processor or by hand.

2 Combine the grated celery, stock, onion, potatoes and cumin in a saucepan. Season with a pinch of salt. Bring to the boil, lower the heat and simmer, partially covered, for 20–25 minutes.

3 Purée the mixture in a blender or food processor until smooth, stir in the reserved sliced celery and allow to cool in a bowl. Chill in the refrigerator for at least 3 hours. Stir in the yogurt just before serving and garnish with the celery leaves.

Grilled aubergine soup

Grilling the aubergines first gives this delicious soup its distinctive, smoky flavour.

SERVES 4

750 g (1½ lb) aubergines

3 tablespoons olive oil

1 onion, chopped

1 carrot, chopped

2 celery sticks, sliced

1 garlic clove, chopped

1.2 litres (2 pints) vegetable stock (see page 52)

2 tablespoons chopped basil

2 tablespoons Parmesan cheese, grated

125 ml (4 fl oz) natural yogurt

salt and pepper

1 Halve the aubergines lengthways and cook under a preheated grill until charred and softened. Allow them to cool, remove any charred patches and chop roughly.

2 In a large, heavy-based saucepan, heat the olive oil and add the onion, carrot, celery, garlic and aubergine. Cover and cook over a low heat for 15 minutes, stirring frequently, until the vegetables are softened.

3 Add the stock, bring the mixture to the boil, cover and simmer gently for 1 hour. Add the basil and allow to cool slightly.

4 Purée the mixture in a blender or food processor until it is very smooth. Return to the saucepan, stir in the Parmesan and yogurt and reheat gently without boiling. Season with salt and pepper to taste, and serve.

friday 9:00 pm **aromatherapy bath**

One of the most common manifestations of stress is insomnia, which can mean not being able to get to sleep or waking in the night and not being able to fall asleep again. Even if you do not suffer from insomnia, you may have a problem with light, restless sleep, which leaves you feeling unrefreshed the next morning. This, in turn, can lead to tension headaches or general aches and pains.

One of the aims of this weekend is to have three deep, restful nights of sleep without recourse to medication and its unwanted side effects. Aromatherapy is a wondrous alternative to sleeping pills and using such a natural remedy means you won't end up feeling drowsy the next day.

You need to take time to wind down at the end of the day, which is why this first evening is so carefully planned, starting with the meditation. Eating a light meal fairly early in the evening also helps. If you feel thirsty later, drink a cup of herbal tea before bed; chamomile with honey and lemon is an ideal bedtime beverage. If you have a tendency towards indigestion, try peppermint tea.

Bathing

An aromatherapy bath is a very good way of slowing down the mind and relaxing the body at the end of the day. This is a bath that has little to do with washing; it is all about succumbing to the pleasures and relaxing powers of the essential oils suspended in the water. Prepare the room in advance to make it as tranquil as possible. The bathroom and towels should be warm. Lighting is also important; keep it as low as possible. Candlelight has a calming effect, and candles scented with relaxing oils are widely available.

Fill the bath with water. It should not be too hot or the oil will simply evaporate. Add 5–10 drops of Sweet dreams oil (see opposite) to the water and mix it in well. Relax in the bath for at least 20 minutes. If you have difficulty unwinding, listen to soft, tranquil music.

After your bath, wrap yourself in a big, warm towel and pat yourself gently with the towel or just wrap yourself in it until it absorbs the water on your body, so that a little of the oil remains on your skin.

Essential oils have therapeutic psychological and physiological effects through their smell and through the skin. They can boost or relax our moods and promote healing in our bodies.

Sweet dreams oil

- 12 drops lavender essential oil
- 8 drops neroli essential oil
- 5 drops rose essential oil

Mix the ingredients together and store in a glass bottle.

friday 10:00 pm **self-massage for sleep**

If you think you may still have trouble sleeping, there are several things you can try. Two or three drops of the Sweet dreams oil (see page 57) on a tissue, placed on your pillow, may help you to unwind if your mind is spinning. If you still feel tense you can give yourself a facial massage. Use half of the mixture and add to it 1 oz (25 ml) of almond oil, grapeseed oil or any other cold-pressed vegetable oil. Shake well and apply it to your face and neck. If you don't mind having oily hair until you shower in the morning, you can also massage the oil into your scalp. You should find this particularly relaxing. Alternatively, use undiluted lavender or neroli oil in a burner and put the burner in the bedroom about half an hour before you go to bed. Be sure to extinguish the burner, though, before climbing into bed.

Self-massage for sleep

This self-massage, using the Sweet dreams oil, will take you only about 5–10 minutes, depending on how slowly you make the strokes. You can do it after your bath or even when you are already in bed, although in that case you will need a large pillow to support your back. Take your time and leave the oil on so it can work all night.

Facial massage

1 Rest your three central fingers of each hand on each eyebrow. Close your eyes lightly and remain in that position for a moment, taking a few deep breaths.

2 Place the middle finger of each hand either side of, and immediately above, the bridge of your nose, between your eyebrows. Now, following the line of the brows, make small circles with your fingers along the length of your brows as far as your temples. When you reach your temples, hold your fingers over them for a moment with a slightly firmer pressure.

Return to the centre of the forehead, this time with your fingers placed very slightly higher, and trace another line out towards your temples again, in the same way.

3 Continue to repeat step 2, each time moving your fingers up slightly more until they are following the

hairline. Then, using the same circular movements, follow the hairline all the way around to the nape of your neck. Repeat this several times.

4 Make the same circular movements from the neck hairline down your neck, with your fingers either side of your spine. Do not place them on the spine itself. You may want to use more pressure here.

5 Use the same movements from the centre of your forehead back across your scalp to the nape of your neck. You may want to use two or three fingers here and make the movement cover a larger area. Finally, using the whole hand, cover the whole of your head, as if you are kneading your scalp.

saturday

8:00 am Yoga	**4:00 pm** Facial massage
9:00 am Breakfast	**6:00 pm** Evening meal
10:00 am Relaxation and meditation	**8:00 pm** Breathing techniques and meditation
12:00 am Lunch	**10:00 pm** Bed
2:00 pm Massage	

saturday 8:00 am **yoga**

Yoga, the ancient Indian 'science of life', deals with physical, mental and spiritual health in its three disciplines of postures, or *asanas*, breathing exercises and meditation. During this relaxation weekend, you will try all of these aspects of yoga.

Yoga is a systematic, gradual process of relaxation and is therefore a perfect technique for this weekend. The physical relaxation that results from the practice of *asanas* and *pranayama* (see page 81) brings with it the release of old stored tensions, often emotional in origin.

The body becomes much more supple and the muscles are stretched and toned without increasing their bulk. Ailments connected with tension and contracted muscles are therefore often considerably relieved by yoga. These include chronic back pain, headaches and migraine. The effect of loosening immobile joints makes yoga particularly helpful for anyone who suffers from arthritis or rheumatism.

saturday 8:00 am **yoga**

Start the day with the practice of a yoga exercise –
before you breakfast or shower. Even if you are not
at your best in the morning, this exercise will wake
up your body and help to focus your mind. It also
works as a massage for the internal organs.

Wear loose clothing and make sure the room
is warm before you start exercising – a cold
atmosphere is not beneficial to stretching muscles.
This exercise is called Salute to the sun and is
traditionally performed in the morning.

Salute to the sun
1 Stand up straight,
looking ahead, palms
together in the prayer
position just in front of
your breastbone. Check
that you are balanced,
with your weight
equally distributed on
both feet and you are
not tensing any area of
your body. Take a few
long, deep breaths.

2 Breathe in deeply
and stretch your arms
up to the ceiling.
Continue the movement
so that your arms move
slightly backwards,
taking your body with
them in a curve. Don't
force this position any
more than feels
comfortable for you.

3 Return to the erect position, still with your arms raised above you and, as you breathe out, bend forwards from your hips, keeping your back straight.

4 Place your hands on the floor. If this isn't possible, hold the backs of your calves or ankles and gently stretch the backs of your legs.

5 Take a deep breath in and bend your left knee, at the same time stretching your right leg out behind you and placing your hands on the floor. Look up to the ceiling.

6 Breathing out, take your left leg back so that you are supported on your hands and feet and your body is in a long straight line.

7 Breathe in, and drop your knees and chest to the floor as you breathe out. Keep your hips raised off the floor.

Yoga teachers often say that if you do only one asana a day, it should be the Sun salutation.

8 As you breathe in, drop your hips to the ground and in a long, snake-like movement, push your upper body through your arms as far as it will go until your back is arched and you are looking up towards the ceiling.

9 As you breathe out, lift your hips up to the ceiling and drop your head so that you make a triangle with the floor.

10 Breathe in, bringing your right knee forwards, leaving your left leg stretched out behind you. Breathe out and, again, look up at the ceiling.

11 Breathe in. As you breathe out, bring your left leg up to meet your right and stretch your legs, your hands flat on the floor or holding the backs of your calves. Keep your head dropped towards the floor. Only stretch as far as feels comfortable and, unless you are very supple, keep your knees bent.

12 Breathe in and very slowly start to lift your body from the waist, arms stretched out in front of you. Go past the upright position so that you lean back, arms behind you.

13 Return to standing and bring your palms together in front of you in the prayer position.

You can repeat this whole dynamic sequence a few times. Those who are experienced at yoga may do so up to 10 times. However, if you are a beginner, you should do it no more than 2 or 3 times at first. You will find that you can stretch further each time you do it.

You may also find it helpful to take one sequence incredibly slowly, holding each of the 12 positions for a few moments and taking a few breaths to relax into them.

When you have finished, take 5 minutes to relax in either of the poses shown opposite.

Pose of the child

This is a very good position to rest in after Salute to the Sun, particularly if your back is not used to so much stretching.

Sit on your heels, back straight. Place your hands behind you on the soles of your feet. Breathe in and bend backwards gently, looking up.

Breathe out and bend slowly forwards until you can place your forehead on the floor. You will have to let go of your feet, and your bottom may come up a little. Allow your arms to lie by your sides and breathe slowly with your eyes closed. After a minute or two of slow, deep breathing, allow your breathing to become shallower, but keep your eyes closed. When you are ready, come up very slowly.

Corpse pose

This pose is so relaxing that you might even fall asleep. Make sure you have something to cover yourself with in this position as otherwise you may begin to feel cold.

Lie on your back with your arms slightly out from your sides with the palms uppermost. Your legs are slightly apart and your feet are relaxed. Now, close your eyes.

Breathe slowly and deeply for 1–2 minutes, concentrating on the breath itself and the sensation of your lungs filling with air. Then breathe naturally for a few more minutes before getting up.

breakfasts

It is best to have breakfast after you have done your yoga session – exercise on a full stomach is not recommended. If you can, drink a herbal infusion rather than ordinary tea or coffee, but if you really can't do without these, try decaffeinated versions – you will sense the benefit when you do your relaxation session later in the morning, and when you go to bed at night.

Keep breakfast simple – perhaps a piece of wholemeal toast or a non-sugary cereal with some fruit and a herbal tea. Have a large glass of fruit juice as well – you could try doing some juicing yourself (see page 22). Look at the few tasty recipes here and opposite for other breakfast ideas.

Drink plenty of filtered or bottled water or more herbal teas throughout the day to keep your fluid intake up and, if you want a snack, have a piece of fruit or some dried fruit and nuts.

Figgy apple
SERVES 1
1 large cooking apple
1 teaspoon clear honey
25 g (1 oz) dried figs
1 teaspoon lemon juice
1 tablespoon apple juice
3 tablespoons low-fat natural yogurt

1 Core the apple and stuff the centre with the honey, figs and the lemon juice.

2 Pour over the apple juice and bake in the oven at 180°C (350°F), Gas Mark 4 for 40 minutes.

3 Serve with the low-fat natural yogurt.

Rather than reaching for your normal cup of tea or coffee in the morning, juice up some exotic fruits or have a herbal tea.

Hot fruit salad

SERVES 1

125 g (4 oz) mixed dried
  fruit, such as apricots,
  prunes,apples, pears
  and figs

150 ml (¼ pint) apple or
  orange juice

25 g (1 oz) walnuts,
  chopped

3 tablespoons low-fat
  natural yogurt (optional)

1 Place all the fruit in
a bowl and add the
juice. Leave to soak
overnight.

2 Pour the contents into
a saucepan and simmer
gently for 10 minutes.

3 Sprinkle with walnuts
and serve with yogurt.

Melons with honey

SERVES 1

¼ small watermelon

¼ small Galia or Ogen
  melon

1 tablespoon clear honey

25 g (1 oz) flaked
  almonds, toasted

1 Remove the seeds
and rind from the
melons and cut them
into small cubes.

2 Gently stir the honey,
into the melon cubes.
Sprinkle with almonds
and serve.

saturday 10:00 am **relaxation and meditation**

After breakfast, you can slowly begin to prepare yourself for the rest of the day, allowing yourself time to digest what you've eaten before you think about your next session.

Dress for the relaxation exercises in clothes that are loose and comfortable. Bear in mind that, during relaxation, your body temperature will drop, so make sure that you are going to be warm enough. Socks are a good idea and put a blanket or sweater nearby in case you begin to feel cold as the session progresses.

There are no secrets to relaxation, and when you try the exercises you may be surprised to find how closely the mind and body track each other. Where one leads, the other will follow; therefore by relaxing one, the other must also relax. However, you have to give yourself the chance to relax – free from interruption. Take the phone off the hook or put on the answer machine and, if anyone is likely to come in and disturb you, put a 'keep out' notice on the other side of the closed door.

There are two ways of completing the relaxation process: you can read through the instructions that follow and remember them, saying them to yourself in your mind; or you can record the whole sequence in advance. The latter method allows you to focus entirely on your body.

Recording your relaxation tape

During relaxation, your mind and body slow down, so you must speak very slowly and calmly. As you will see, there is a good deal of repetition in what you say – this helps you to focus your mind. Leave pauses between each instruction – it is a good idea to take at least one long, deep breath between each sentence, with a longer pause between each individual instruction. In some places, for example where you have to repeat a series of procedures, you will have to leave enough of a pause for you to attend to these on the tape.

You may not be able to focus on one part of your body immediately, and it is important to give yourself plenty of time. Don't put any modulation into your voice; it may sound boring to you as you record it, but you don't want any surprises or excitement during relaxation!

The whole tape, with pauses, should take approximately 30–40 minutes, but you can make it longer if you wish. You can estimate how long you need by reading the instructions aloud before you start to record them.

Music – to play or not to play?

Some people like to play music in the background. However, this can be a distraction. You start listening to the music instead of focusing on your body. There are tapes available that feature music designed for relaxation and, when you have practised the technique for a while, you may find one of these makes an interesting change.

Yogic sleep

There are many ways one can approach the relaxation process, and the one given here is very loosely based on the yoga *nidra* or relaxation technique. *Nidra* means 'yogic sleep', but you are, in fact, very much aware and carry your awareness around your body, focusing on each area in turn. Bearing this in mind, it is important not to fall asleep – so make sure the room is warm but not stuffy before you start. Put the tape within easy reach so you don't have to get up to switch it on after the preparation.

Preparing for relaxation

Lie on the floor in the Corpse pose (see page 65), covering yourself with a blanket or towel if you feel cold. Take three long, slow, deep breaths, concentrating on the exhalation so that your body feels quite empty before you breathe in again.

Starting at your toes, and working up through your legs and body, tense each group of muscles in turn, then relax them and move on to the next. Do not expect your muscles to relax completely at this stage, simply become aware of them. You will need to move some parts of your body, such as your shoulders and your head, by rolling or rotating rather than tensing. But even so these are all very slight movements.

When you have become aware of all parts of your body, simply lie still for a few moments, still with legs slightly apart and hands by your sides, and then switch on the tape.

saturday 10:00 am **relaxation and meditation**

Relaxation exercise

Focus your awareness on your left foot. Become aware of this foot. Take your awareness to your toes.

- Become aware of your big toe. Feel your big toe soften and relax. Become aware of your second toe. Feel it soften and relax. Become aware of your third toe. Feel it soften and relax. Become aware of your fourth toe. Feel it soften and relax. Become aware of your little toe. Feel it soften and relax. All your toes are soft and relaxed.
- Take your awareness into the sole of the foot. It is relaxing. Your left sole is relaxed.
- Take your awareness into your left heel. It is relaxing. Your left heel is relaxed.
- Take your awareness into the top of your foot. It is relaxing. The top of your foot is relaxed.
- Become aware of your left ankle. It is relaxing. Your left ankle is relaxed.
- Become aware of your left calf, the calf muscle, the shin, the knee. Your left calf is relaxing. It has become relaxed. The shin is relaxing. It has become relaxed. Your left knee is relaxing. It has become relaxed.
- Let your awareness flow up towards your thigh. Feel the muscles in the front of your thigh relaxing. They are relaxed.
- Feel the muscles in the back of your thigh relaxing. They are relaxed.
- Let your awareness travel higher, up into your left buttock. Feel your buttock muscles relaxing. They are relaxed.
- The whole of your left leg, from your toes to your buttocks, is now relaxed.

Now repeat the whole sequence on the right leg.

Take your awareness into your abdomen.

- Become aware of your abdomen. Become aware of how your abdomen rises and falls as you breathe. Become aware of the rising and falling. Your abdomen is relaxing. Your breathing is relaxing. Your abdomen is relaxed.
- Focus your awareness on your pelvic area. Become aware of the sexual organs, the bladder, the colon. Feel them all relaxing. The whole pelvic area is relaxed.
- Become aware of your back. Feel your lower back, your middle back, your upper back against the floor. Feel your lower back, your middle back, your upper back relaxing. The whole of your back is relaxed.
- Become aware of your chest. Become aware of it rising and falling as you breathe. Feel your lungs expand and contract as you breathe. Feel your lungs soften and relax. Feel your chest soften and relax. The whole of your chest is relaxed.

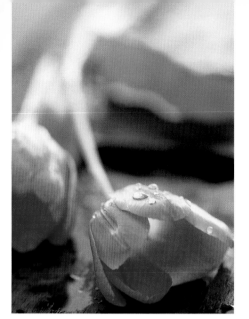

Take your awareness into your left hand.

- Become aware of your fingers. Become aware of your little finger. Feel it soften and relax. Become aware of your next finger. Feel it soften and relax. Become aware of your middle finger. Feel it soften and relax. Become aware of your index finger. Feel it soften and relax. Become aware of your thumb. Feel it soften and relax. All your fingers are relaxed.
- Become aware of your palm. Your palm is relaxing. It is relaxed.
- Become aware of the back of your hand. The back of your hand is relaxing. It is relaxed.
- Become aware of your wrist. Your wrist is relaxing. It is relaxed.
- Become aware of your forearm, front and back. It is relaxing. Your whole forearm is relaxed.
- Become aware of your elbow. Your elbow is relaxing. It is relaxed.
- Become aware of your upper arm, front and back. It is relaxing. Your upper arm is relaxed.
- Become aware of your left shoulder. It is relaxing. Your shoulder is relaxed. The whole of your left arm is relaxed.

Repeat on your right arm.

Take your awareness upwards to your neck.

- Become aware of your throat and neck. They are relaxing. Your throat and neck are relaxed.
- Become aware of your face. Become aware of your jaw, your chin, your cheeks, your nose, your lips. They are all relaxing. Inside your mouth, your tongue, your lips, all are relaxing. Become aware of your left eye, the eyelid, the eyebrow. They are all relaxing. Become aware of your right eye, the eyelid, the eyebrow. They are all relaxing. Become aware of your forehead. It is relaxing. Your forehead is relaxed. The whole of your face is relaxed.
- Become aware of your ears. Your ears are relaxing. They are relaxed.
- Become aware of your scalp. The whole of your scalp is relaxing. Your whole head is relaxed.
- Become aware of a point at the top of your head. It is relaxing. The top of your head is relaxed and is opening like a flower.
- Golden light is pouring into the top of your head. It is pouring through your head, down through your body, through your arms, through your legs. The golden light is bringing peace and healing to your whole body. Be aware of your whole body pulsing with golden light.
- Feel the top of your head close, like a flower closing its petals for the night. The top of your head is closed but your body is still filled with golden light. Feel the golden light stream through your body on your breath. Feel how light and weightless your body is on the floor.
- Become aware of the lightness of your breath. Become aware of your breath coming into your body. Become aware of your breath leaving your body. Be aware of your breath for a time.
- Take your awareness into the rest of your body. Become aware of your arms, your legs, your back, your chest, your abdomen. Be aware of it breathing on the floor.

On completion

Lie on the floor for at least 5 minutes afterwards. If you get up too soon, you may feel dizzy. So, lie on the floor and gradually come back to normal consciousness. You may want to lie on the bed or even take a short nap. Do whatever you feel and spend the time until lunch as quietly as possible.

lunches

Lunch will be the main meal of the day for the weekend, so do enjoy it. Have two courses, chosen from the following selection and give yourself plenty of time to savour the food.

Greek salad with tahini dressing

SERVES 1

½ small green pepper, deseeded, and sliced

½ small cucumber, cut into thin batons

175 g (6 oz) tomatoes, cut into thin wedges

½ small onion, thinly sliced

8 small black olives, halved

50 g (2 oz) feta cheese

wholemeal pitta bread, to serve

TAHINI DRESSING

1 tablespoon tahini paste

2 tablespoons low-fat natural yogurt

1 tablespoon water

1 tablespoon chopped parsley

1 small garlic clove, crushed

salt and pepper

1 Place the green pepper, cucumber, tomatoes, onion and olives in a salad bowl.

2 To make the dressing, spoon the tahini paste into a small bowl and slowly beat in the yogurt, thinning with water if necessary. Stir in the parsley and garlic. Season with salt and pepper.

3 Pour the dressing over the vegetables and toss well.

4 Cut the feta cheese into small cubes and sprinkle them over the salad. Serve with warm pitta bread.

Chicken salad with tarragon and orange

SERVES 2

½ chicken, with giblets, about 750 g (1½ lb)

½ onion

grated rind and juice of 1 orange

½ tablespoon chopped tarragon

1 bay leaf

150 ml (¼ pint) water

1 tablespoon olive oil

½–1 tablespoon wine vinegar

salt and pepper

mixed salad leaves, to serve (optional)

TO GARNISH

1 small orange, peeled and diced

½ carton mustard and cress

1 Put the chicken giblets, onion, orange rind and juice, tarragon and bay leaf into a large saucepan.

2 Put the chicken in the saucepan, pour in the water and sprinkle with salt and pepper. Cover, bring to the boil and simmer for about 45 minutes, basting several times until the chicken is cooked.

3 Lift out the chicken and leave to cool. Discard the bay leaf, giblets and onion. Measure the stock.

4 Boil the stock until it has reduced to 300 ml (½ pint). Leave to cool, then chill in the refrigerator.

5 When the chicken is cold, take the meat off the bones, discarding the skin and bones. Cut the meat into bite-size pieces and place in a mixing bowl.

6 To make the dressing, when the stock is chilled, remove the layer of fat from the top. Reheat the stock gently to thin it, stir in the oil, and add the vinegar; then season with salt and pepper to taste.

7 Pour this dressing over the chicken and toss well. Serve at once or cover and chill until required.

8 To serve, turn into a serving dish and garnish with orange slices and cress. Serve the salad on a bed of lettuce, if liked.

Butterfly prawns with basil

SERVES 1

250 g (8 oz) uncooked king prawns, shells on

75 g (3 oz) salad leaves

50 g (2 oz) cherry tomatoes, halved

few sprigs of basil

MARINADE

2 tablespoons lemon juice

2 tablespoons olive oil

½ garlic clove, crushed

1 teaspoon chopped basil

salt and pepper

DRESSING

1 tablespoon tarragon vinegar

½ teaspoon finely grated lemon rind

¼ teaspoon Dijon mustard

½ tablespoon chopped tarragon

3 tablespoons olive oil

few sprigs basil

1 To prepare the prawns, remove the heads and carefully cut them almost in half lengthways, leaving the tail end intact. Remove the dark vein from the back. Place the prawns in a single layer in a shallow dish.

2 Mix all the marinade ingredients and pour it over the prawns. Cover and leave for 1 hour.

3 Remove the prawns and arrange them on a rack over a grill pan. Cook under a hot grill for 3–4 minutes until they have curled and are bright pink.

4 Arrange the salad leaves and tomatoes on a plate and scatter with the basil. Then arrange the prawns on top.

5 Shake all the dressing ingredients together in a jar. Pour it over the salad; serve.

Frozen yogurt with melon

SERVES 4

large Ogen or Charentais melon

300 ml (½ pint) low-fat natural yogurt

1 Halve the melon and scoop out all the seeds. Scoop the flesh into a food processor or blender and process until smooth.

2 Mix the melon purée with the yogurt.

3 Transfer to a shallow freezer container and freeze until firm.

4 Remove from the freezer about 20 minutes before serving. Serve in scoops.

Hot chicken and walnut salad

SERVES 1

50 g (2 oz) mange tout, halved

125 g (4 oz) salad leaves

½ red onion, thinly sliced

1 skinless chicken breast fillet

2 tablespoons olive oil

1 tablespoon walnut oil

1 garlic clove, crushed

1 tablespoon wine vinegar

25 g (1 oz) walnut pieces

pared rind of ½ lemon, thinly sliced

½ teaspoon soft light brown sugar

salt and pepper

parsley sprigs, roughly chopped, to garnish

1 Bring a saucepan of water to the boil, add the mange tout and blanch for 1 minute. Drain thoroughly.

2 Tear the salad leaves into bite-size pieces and arrange on a plate, with the mange tout and the onion.

3 Cut the chicken breast into thick slices. Using a rolling pin, flatten the slices between two sheets of greaseproof paper or clingfilm to make thin medallions.

4 Heat the olive oil in a frying pan or wok. Add the chicken pieces, a few at a time, and cook over a high heat for 2 minutes, turning once, until lightly browned and cooked through.

5 Add the walnut oil to the pan, stir in the remaining ingredients and season with salt and pepper. Heat through, stirring, then return the chicken to the pan.

6 Toss the chicken in just enough of the hot dressing to coat, then pile the chicken mixture in the centre of the salad leaves. Garnish with parsley and serve.

Spiced pears

SERVES 4

4 large firm pears

½ lemon

16 cloves

½ cinnamon stick

300 ml (½ pint) apple juice

2 tablespoons redcurrant jelly

4 orange slices

4 small bay leaves, to decorate

1 Peel the pears, leaving the stalks intact. Rub them all over with the lemon half to prevent discoloration.

2 Stud each pear with four cloves. Stand them upright in a pan and add the cinnamon stick, apple juice and enough water just to cover the pears.

3 Bring to the boil and simmer gently until the pears are just tender. Leave to cool.

4 Put 2 tablespoons of the cooking liquid into a small pan with the redcurrant jelly. Bubble briskly for about 1 minute until the jelly has dissolved.

5 Place an orange slice on each plate. Drain the pears with a slotted spoon and sit one on top of each orange slice.

6 Spoon a little of the redcurrant glaze over each pear and decorate with a bay leaf.

Whole strawberry ice cream

SERVES 4

3 egg yolks

1 tablespoon redcurrant jelly

1 tablespoon red vermouth

300 ml (½ pint) low-fat natural yogurt

375 g (12 oz) ripe strawberries, hulled

4–6 strawberries, with stalks, halved, to decorate

1 Put the egg yolks into a food processor or blender with the redcurrant jelly, red vermouth, yogurt and half the strawberries. Blend together until smooth.

2 Transfer the mixture to a shallow freezerproof container and freeze until the mixture starts to harden around the edges.

3 Tip the ice cream into a bowl and beat to break up the ice crystals. Chop all the remaining hulled strawberries and mix them into the ice cream. Return to the container and freeze until firm.

4 Remove the ice cream from the freezer about 20 minutes before serving. Serve in scoops, decorated with strawberry halves.

All these delicious desserts are full of vitamin C, so you can treat yourself and know that you're doing your body good, too.

saturday 2:00 pm **massage**

Delay the massage until you have had a chance to digest your lunch. The ultimate treat is to have a professional massage – and it is particularly relaxing if aromatherapy oils are used. Look for a qualified therapist at your local gym, swimming pool or sports centre, and make sure you book your appointment well in advance. Some therapists will even come to you. This is the best possible option; after you have had your massage you can simply relax at home. However, you don't need to find a professional. You can learn to give a massage very easily and, if you learn with a friend, you can take turns. There are a number of weekend courses available that will teach you the basics.

The massage described here is quite straightforward and very relaxing, particularly if you use oils. Oils will also help your hands slide smoothly over the skin, but always take time to warm them in your hands before you start. As with relaxation, it is important to keep warm, so make sure the room is warmer than you would normally have it, and that there are plenty of towels to cover up any parts of your body not being massaged. Cold muscles become tense, which defeats the whole point of the massage.

Make sure you aren't going to be disturbed and don't talk during the massage – unless it is to ask about the massage – as this is a disturbance in itself. When you give the massage, wear loose, comfortable clothes and take off any jewellery. You can either have a background of silence or play soothing music very quietly. Do the massage on the floor or a hard bed.

Try to trust your instincts when you give a massage and rely on your own sense of touch. You will soon get to know the feel of tense muscles that need to be released. Check at the start that you are using the right pressure for your partner – not so vigorous that it becomes painful or so light that it doesn't get to the root of the problem.

Never massage:

- anyone with a heart condition
- broken or infected skin or varicose veins
- joints swollen by rheumatism or arthritis.

The body massage

The first person to be massaged should lie face down on the floor (with a towel underneath) or on a bed. Cover them with towels. In this massage attend to the upper body; it is the back, shoulders and neck that are usually the centres of tension, so you will be concentrating on the areas that need to relax most. However, you can continue and do a whole body massage if you wish. In this case, it is better if you start with the lower body and massage the legs first, then work up to the back, finishing, as here, with the neck and shoulders.

As the aim here is to get you or your partner to relax, you may find it most comfortable when lying face down to turn your head to one side. Turn your head during the massage or your neck may get tense on one side. Alternatively, you can put a pillow under your forehead to raise the head off the floor while maintaining a straight spine.

1 Make sure your partner is lying comfortably face down and uncover the back. Warm the oil in your hands and place them flat on the lower back, with your fingers pointing towards the neck. Leave your hands still for a moment to let your partner get used to your touch.

With your hands on either side of the spine – not on the spine itself – gently glide up the back, spreading the oil as you go.

2 When you get to the top of the back, move out to the shoulders and then gently along the sides. Repeat several times, keeping your hands flat throughout, in a slow stroking movement. In massage technique, this is known as effleurage.

3 Starting again at the base of the spine, work up the back, with the hands either side of the spine. This time, make little circles, using your thumbs only. You can apply more pressure in this movement, and it is a very good way of releasing tension knots. However, check with your partner that you are not using too much pressure; it should not hurt. Repeat several times. Remember, never massage the spine itself. Always work to each side of it.

4 Knead the neck muscles, using both hands in the same way as you would knead bread. Knead gently here as these muscles can often be very tense.

5 Place one hand on top of the other at the neck. Make a figure-of-eight movement across the upper back, using the weight of your body to iron out the tension. Your hands circle the first shoulder, then move diagonally across the back to circle the opposite shoulder blade, returning to the centre of the back and circling the first shoulder again. Repeat this several times.

6 Move around to your partner's head and, with your fingers pointing down the back, make a long stroking movement all the way down the back, placing your hands on either side of the spine. Use your body weight to help release tense muscles. At the base of the spine, move your hands out across the tops of the buttocks, then up the sides back to the shoulders. Repeat this step several times, gradually making the pressure lighter with each repetition.

7 Starting at the base of the spine, and using the middle finger of each hand in turn, stroke the whole length of the spine as far as the neck. Lift the finger off at the top and repeat with the middle finger of the other hand. Each time, the pressure becomes increasingly lighter, until it is as light as a feather.

8 Ask your partner to turn over and cover them with towels, leaving the neck and shoulders uncovered. Warm some more of the oil in your hands. Lay them flat on each side of the upper chest and leave them there for a few moments.

9 With a long, firm, stroking movement, take your hands to the centre of the chest, and then out to the sides.

10 Continue the stroking movements under the shoulders and back up to the neck, pulling out the muscles as you do so. This should help the back and neck to lie flatter on the floor.

11 Using the circular thumb movement you used on the back, move your hands across the upper chest. Start just below the collarbone, working outwards from the centre. Repeat this several times, each time moving down gradually.

12 Place your hands, fingertips pointing downwards, on the upper chest. Move them out smoothly across the chest, over the upper arms, and up over the shoulders back to the chest. Repeat this several times. Place the hands on the upper chest and hold them there for a minute or two. Cover your partner with the towels and leave him/her to relax for a few moments.

Relaxing massage oil

- 10 drops lavender essential oil
- 10 drops geranium essential oil
- 5 drops jasmine essential oil

Place the ingredients in 50 ml (2 fl oz) of carrier oil, such as almond, grapeseed or any cold-pressed vegetable oil. Mix well and store in a dark glass bottle.

saturday 4:00 pm **facial massage**

The facial

It may comes as a surprise to realize that a lot of tension is stored in the muscles of the face. Frown lines are an obvious example, but rigid jaws, pursed lips and staring eyes are other tell-tale signs. A facial massage releases this tension and leaves your face looking relaxed, and therefore younger. Also, because the massage stimulates circulation to the face, your complexion should be toned and glowing by the end of this session.

1 Begin by cleansing your face thoroughly. Put on a light moisturizer, covering your throat and face with a thin layer.

2 Place your hands at your jawline so that your middle fingers are resting on your jaw, just below your ears. Making small circles with the middle fingers, work your way gradually to the centre of your chin. Keep your jaw relaxed while you do this. Do this 3 times.

3 Return to the starting position, as described in step 2, but this time make gentle pinching movements along the length of the jawline. Repeat 5 times.

4 To release tension in your forehead, place your middle fingers between your eyebrows and make small circles as you work your way out along the eyebrows towards your temples. Repeat this several times, each time beginning a fraction higher up the forehead until you reach the hairline.

5 Hold your earlobes between your thumbs and forefingers. Gently rub the lobes between your fingers and thumbs. Now work your way along the outer edge of your ears, gently rubbing all the way, until you reach the top. Repeat 5 times.

6 To stimulate the eye area, begin with your middle fingers on the inner corners of each eyebrow. Making little tapping movements as you go, work your way along the eyebrow, then follow the eye socket round, across the top of your cheekbone and up the sides of your nose. Circle your eyes 5 times.

7 Starting again at the inner corners of your eyebrows, squeeze along the whole length of the eyebrows using your thumbs and forefingers. Then move to your temples and, using your forefingers and middle fingers together, rub gently in a circular motion. Repeat 5 times.

8 Starting at the base of your nose, press your three middle fingers below your cheekbones, gradually working out in a line towards your ears.

9 Use all your fingers to pat your face gently in a ripple effect, tracing the outline of your face from your forehead, out past your ears to your jawline and into the centre of your chin. Then let your fingers play over the whole of your face in a gentle tapping rhythm for 2 minutes.

10 Finally, rub the palms of your hands together and place them on your face so that the heels of your hands are resting on your cheekbones and your eyes are covered. Hold this position for 2 minutes.

saturday 8:00 pm
breathing techniques and meditation

Breathing relaxation

In yoga, ill health is regarded as the product of imbalances and blockages in the flow of energy, or *prana*, through the body. *Prana* is believed to permeate everything in the world around us and, in the human body, it flows in channels called *nadis*; similarly, in Chinese medicine energy or *chi* flows through meridians in the body.

The practice of *pranayama* takes the form of breathing exercises. Unlike circulation or digestion, we can consciously control our breathing, and this acts as a link between the conscious and the unconscious parts of our bodies.

Pranayama exercises improve oxygen intake, purification and circulation of the blood and lymph, increasing the flow of oxygen to every cell in the body. These exercises also improve mental alertness, concentration and creativity, as well as being deeply relaxing, producing a sense of calm and serenity; furthermore, they can dispel tension when used at times of stress, when breathing typically becomes fast and shallow.

The *pranayama* breathing exercises, together with many of the *asanas* or yoga postures, also open the chest, strengthening the respiratory muscles and stretching out the lungs. This is beneficial for respiratory disorders such as sinusitis and hay fever, as well as asthma and bronchitis. Given the invigorating effect of improved circulation and posture, the body's immune system becomes more efficient, improving resistance to disease.

In both of the breathing exercises that follow, focus your attention on your breath and try to observe its progress through your body.

Meditation

The breathing exercises are very relaxing and slow the body down considerably. This puts you in the ideal state for meditation. So, as soon as you are ready, do your second meditation session, choosing one of the methods on page 51.

Deep breathing

This exercise helps establish a slower, deeper breathing rhythm, which in turn slows the heart rate and aids relaxation.

1 Lie on the floor, placing your hands on your abdomen, fingertips touching. Take a long, slow breath in through your nose, counting to five. Your lungs and abdomen will expand, making your fingertips part.

2 Hold a deep breath for the count of 5. Then, very slowly, this time on a count of 10, exhale through your mouth. Feel your fingertips touch again and keep on going, trying to empty your body completely of air. Repeat the whole sequence 10 times.

Alternate nostril breathing

For this exercise, sit comfortably on the floor, legs crossed, keeping your spine straight. Alternatively, kneel on the floor, sitting back on your heels, or sit on a chair. Choose whichever position is the most comfortable.

1 Close your eyes and breathe in. Lift your right hand up so it is level with your face and, using your thumb, close your right nostril. Exhale slowly through your left nostril, then breathe in again.

2 Now close your left nostril with your middle finger. Exhale and inhale through your right nostril. Repeat the whole sequence 10 times.

sunday

8:00 am Yoga, relaxation and meditation	**4:00 pm** Meditation
9:00 am Breakfast	**6:00 pm** Evening meal
11:00 am Acupressure	**8:00 pm** Aromatherapy bath
1:00 pm Lunch	**10:00 pm** Bed
3:00 pm Aromatherapy facial	

sunday 8:00 am
yoga, relaxation and meditation

You should be feeling much more relaxed and well rested than you did when you woke up on Saturday. As yesterday, the day starts with a yoga session. Begin with Salute to the sun on pages 62–63 – repeating between 3 and 10 times, depending on how experienced you are and how fit and supple you feel. Then proceed to the following postures. As with all yoga exercises, do them slowly, and do not put any unnecessary strain on your body. If you feel at all uncomfortable or have any pain, come out of the posture, rest and then move on to something else.

Yoga postures
The postures that follow stretch, stimulate and bring into balance various parts of the body. The first focuses on stretching the back while the second stretches the front of the body.

The triangle

This sideways bend benefits the spine and balances muscle groups.

1 Stand with your feet together, keeping your back stretched and looking straight ahead. Your body should feel alert yet relaxed. Place your feet on the floor 60–90 cm (24–36 inches) apart, then turn your right foot so that it points outwards at a right angle to your body. Your left foot should point slightly to the right.

Breathe in deeply and raise your arms to shoulder height, parallel to the floor. As you breathe out, bend to the right, placing your right hand on the thigh of your right leg, and sliding it down your calf as far as you can towards the floor. Do not twist your body as you slide down; your hips should be facing directly forwards.

2 Raise your left arm so that your fingers point to the ceiling and your palm faces forwards. Turn your head so you are looking up at your hand. Feel a long stretch down your left side and between your right and left hands. Take at least 3 long breaths in this position, 10 if you can.

Breathing in, slide your right arm back up, dropping your left arm until you are facing forwards again. Repeat on the left. Do 3 stretches on each side.

The cobra

This posture stretches the front of the body and compresses the spine. The whole movement should be done slowly, with controlled movements, both while raising the body off the floor and coming down again.

1 Lie face down on the floor, legs together, toes pointing away from you. Place your hands flat on the floor, parallel with your chest. Your forehead should be touching the floor.

2 Breathe in deeply and slowly start to raise your head, feeling a stretch through the back of your neck. Look at the floor to avoid tension in your neck. Breathe out.

3 Breathe in again and continue to lift your head. As you do so your chest should come up from the floor. Bring your arms in front of you and use them to support your body as you lift the whole ribcage off the floor. Look directly in front of you. When you have lifted as high as you can without undue strain, press down on your hands, breathe out and, if you can, hold this position for several breaths.

Breathe in deeply and return to the starting position, going through each of the stages you did on the way up. Rest for a moment and repeat the sequence once more if you feel that you can.

Shoulder stand and the plough

The shoulder stand increases energy flow, improves the circulation and stimulates the thyroid gland. It also promotes body awareness. The plough is another inverted posture, or *asana*, that calms the mind but also stimulates the body.
Caution: Do not do the shoulder stand or the plough if you are menstruating or have back problems. If you suffer from hypertension (high blood pressure) or neck problems, check with your doctor before trying these postures.

1 Lie on your back, arms by your sides, and breathe in as you bend your knees to your chest. Breathe out and straighten your legs as far as comfortable, taking them further back so your hips start to come off the floor.

2 Use your hands to support your back and push yourself a little higher. The aim is to straighten your legs so that they are completely perpendicular, while you are resting on your shoulders.

3 If you are able to get your legs into a vertical position, hold this pose, breathing slowly, for 1 to 3 minutes. You can

stretch and flex your feet in this position to help your legs relax.

However, you may find this difficult at first and it may be more comfortable to leave them at a 45 degree angle to your body. If so, go on to step 4.

4 Take your legs over your head and, if you can, place your feet on the floor behind you, toes curled under and legs straight. This is the plough position.

When you are secure in this position, place your arms behind you, flat on the floor. Take several deep breaths in this position.

You can now return to the shoulder stand and go back to the floor by reversing the first two steps, continuing very slowly. Alternatively, roll your spine down slowly back to the floor from the plough position.

sunday 8:00 am
yoga, relaxation and meditation

The fish

This posture opens the chest and compresses the vertebrae in the spine, so it acts as a counter position to the shoulder stand.
Caution: Do not do this exercise if you have neck problems. If you suffer from high blood pressure, avoid putting your head on the floor in step 2, as there is a vital pressure point at the top of the head. As an alternative, you can bend your head back until it is about 2.5 cm (1 inch) from the floor.

1 Lie on your back with your legs held together in front of you and your toes stretching away. Now, raise your back off the ground.

2 Arch your back, while supporting yourself on your elbows with your lower arms and palms of your hands flat on the floor. Lower the top of your head to the floor. Hold this position and take several deep breaths.
   Slide the back of your head and then your neck back down to the floor. Relax for a few moments.

Relaxation and meditation

At the end of this longer yoga session, spend at least 5 minutes in one of the relaxation poses, either the Corpse pose or the Pose of the child (see page 65). You will now be in an ideal frame of mind for meditation. Meditate for up to 20 minutes and, if you wish, do the relaxation and meditation session (see pages 70–71).

sunday 11:00 am **acupressure**

Acupressure

This tactile therapy gives many of the benefits of acupuncture with the great bonuses that you can do it yourself and no needles are involved. As with all forms of Chinese medicine, the underlying principles relate to the smooth flow of the body's energy, or *chi*, which is vital to health and well being. *Chi* travels around the body in channels known as meridians. If the energy flow is blocked as a result of physical or emotional disturbances, the body is thrown off balance. By restoring the flow of *chi*, health is restored.

Stress is all too likely to affect the flow of *chi*. Such disruptions to energy flow can result in many physical symptoms and ailments, including headaches, digestive upsets and insomnia.

The right pressure

You can use your thumb or fingertip to apply pressure on a particular acupressure point. Use a firm, constant pressure with the finger or thumb held straight on the point. Keep the pressure even for 2 minutes.

There are two main pressure points for general stress relief, both of which are easy to locate yourself.

1 Foot pressure point

This is on the top of the foot, about halfway up. It is the point where the bones between the first and second toes meet.

2 Hand pressure point

This is located in the web between the thumb and forefinger on the back of the hand.

3 Head pressure point

This is the point at the centre on the very top of the head. **Caution:** Do not put pressure on this point if you have high blood pressure.

4 Headaches

The foot pressure point, which is for general stress relief, is also good for banishing headaches. Another point is located 4 finger-widths below the knee, outside the tibia.

5 Insomnia

The pressure point for insomnia is located 4 finger-widths above the ankle bone, on the inside of the leg, close to the tibia. **Caution:** Never apply pressure to this point during pregnancy.

6 Indigestion

Applying pressure to this point will help relieve heartburn and nausea. Find the point where the bones meet between the second and the third toes on the top of the foot.

sunday 3:00 pm **aromatherapy facial**

Aromatherapy hair treatment

Before you start your facial, apply an aromatherapy treatment to your hair. When you have made up the recipe, apply the mixture to your whole head, massaging well into your scalp and making sure that all of your hair is coated in oil. Wrap a towel around your hair and then move on to the facial. Leave the oils on for at least as long as it takes to do the facial, although you could leave the treatment on overnight and wash your hair when you shower tomorrow morning.

Cleansing masks

For dry skin
Put 2 teaspoons of clear, runny honey in a bowl. Add 2 drops of lavender oil and 2 drops of rose. Blend well.

For normal to oily skin
Put 2 teaspoons of natural yogurt in a bowl and add 2 drops of lemon oil and 2 drops of cypress oil. Blend well.

Facial toners

Pour 50 ml (2 fl oz) of bottled water into a small, clean mist sprayer.

For normal to dry skin
Add 4 drops of lavender oil, 4 drops of rose oil and 2 drops of geranium. Shake well to mix.

For oily skin
Add 4 drops of lavender, 4 drops of vetivert and 2 drops of bergamot. Shake well to mix.

Spray over your face and throat with your eyes closed.

Essential oil skin conditioners

The recipe is for a larger quantity than you will need for just one application; so store it in a glass bottle for use next time. The essential oils are blended in 50 ml (2 fl oz) of carrier oil. Use cold-pressed vegetable oil or if you have dry or problem skin try using calendula or wheatgerm oil.

For dry skin

Rose	10 drops
Lavender	10 drops
Sandalwood	5 drops

For normal to oily skin

Lemon	10 drops
Lavender	10 drops
Cypress	5 drops

For mature skin

Frankincense	10 drops
Neroli	10 drops
Rose	5 drops

Essential oil hair treatments

Add the following essential oils to 50 ml (2 fl oz) of any cold-pressed vegetable oil.

For greasy hair

Cedarwood	10 drops
Lavender	10 drops
Grapefruit	5 drops

For dry and damaged hair

Rosewood	10 drops
Lavender	10 drops
Sandalwood	5 drops

This facial deep cleanses and rejuvenates the skin. You can buy products over the counter that have essential oils added or make those described opposite using aromatherapy oils and other natural ingredients. You may want to apply the treatments to both your hair and your hands at the same time.

1 Begin by cleansing your skin thoroughly. Use a cleanser that you remove with water. You can then exfoliate your skin with a mini-loofah, specifically designed for use on your face, while your skin is still wet. Use gentle, small circular movements, avoiding your eye area and concentrating on your forehead, nose, chin and cheeks. Rinse well with clean water.

2 Tone your skin with floral water. If you are using a proprietary brand, look for one that is alcohol free. You can make your own facial toner (see opposite).

3 Apply a cleansing mask to your face and throat, avoiding your eye area. Use any leftover mask on the backs of your hands. You can either buy a proprietary cleansing mask or make your own, according to skin type (see opposite).

To make a compress for your eyes, put 1 drop of chamomile oil into 1 litre (1¾ pints) cold water. Mix well.

Soak 2 cotton wool pads in this and squeeze out any excess liquid. Place over your eyes. Relax with the mask and compresses in place for 10 minutes. Then, rinse off with cool water.

4 Apply an essential oil skin conditioner (see opposite), according to skin type. You can use these as night-time moisturizers on a regular basis, too. Apply the mixture to your face and throat. Leave it on for at least 20 minutes, then rinse off. Or, if you prefer, you can leave this on while you are in the bath or even all night.

After your facial and hair treatment you should be feeling very relaxed. This is a perfect time for your afternoon meditation.

And after dinner round off your relaxing weekend with a slumber-inducing aromatherapy bath (see pages 56–57).

energizing
weekend

The Weekend

This is the weekend for anyone who feels they are continually under par, performing at 80 per cent or less of their full capacity. This weekend should be a tonic that puts you back on form, boosts your immune system and raises energy levels. If you wake up feeling tired and you would rather feel as if you were ready for anything, or if you are continually suffering from colds and flu, and never feel completely healthy, help is at hand.

friday

7:00 pm
Autogenic training

7:30 pm
Evening meal

10:00 pm
Autogenic training

saturday

8:00 am
Autogenic training

8:30 am
Warm-up and stretches

9:30 am
High-energy drink or muesli

10:00 am
Salt scrub

10:30 am
Aromatherapy

11:30 am
Autogenic training

12:00 am
Lunch

3:00 pm
Ayurveda

5:00 pm
Autogenic training

6:00 pm
Evening meal

10:00 pm
Autogenic training

sunday

8:00 am
Autogenic training

8:30 am
Warm-up and stretches

9:30 am
High-energy drink or muesli

10:00 am
Shower (with optional salt scrub)

10:30 am
Reflexology

11:00 am
Autogenic training

12:00 am
Lunch

3:00 pm
Chi kung

5:00 pm
Autogenic training

6:00 pm
Evening meal

10:00 pm
Autogenic training

7:00 pm
Autogenic training
7:30 pm
Evening meal
10:00 pm
Autogenic training

friday 7:00 pm **autogenic training**

Autogenic training is a form of relaxation that verges on meditation. This technique can be used both as a long-term relaxation therapy and as a quick defuser of stressful situations.

Ideally, autogenic training is a technique that should be learned with a therapist, who will take you through several stages over a period of weeks. Unfortunately there are still relatively few autogenic training teachers, so the bare bones of the technique are described here. You will probably find that you will not need to go any further than stage 3 during the weekend.

This is most definitely not a race. If you really feel that you are falling into a relaxed state very quickly at the start of each session, you could try proceeding to the next stage, but it doesn't matter if you are still on stage 1 by the end of the weekend.

Each session takes a matter of minutes. It becomes slightly longer at each stage. You can repeat each stage regularly throughout the weekend as you advance, but make sure you do at least 4 sessions a day. The best times are first thing in the morning, mid-morning just before lunch, mid-afternoon, just before supper and last thing at night in bed (for a great night's sleep). The minimum number and times of the sessions are given in the schedule for each day's activities.

You can sit or lie down during autogenic training, whichever you prefer. While you are learning the technique, it is a good idea to find a quiet room where you will not be disturbed. But, once you become more adept, you will find you can use it any time any where as an instant way of relieving stress – in the office, while travelling or before an exam or an interview, for example.

As with all forms of meditation and relaxation, you should focus your mind quietly, without worrying if you find your mind drifting away on other thoughts. Just bring your mind gently back to where it is supposed to be. Autogenic training focuses on various parts of the body in turn and the sense of physical relaxation induces a mental relaxation. Focus your mind on the specific physical area at each stage. Don't worry if you don't feel heaviness initially – this will come. Don't worry either if you feel other physical sensations, such as numbness or floating. This is perfectly normal.

Adopt the position
When you practise in bed or on the floor, lie on your back with your arms at your sides, allowing your limbs to fall naturally. If you are sitting, make sure your back is well supported and sit up straight, your feet flat on the floor and your hands resting on your thighs. Begin with some quiet time breathing slowly and deeply. When you have finished the session, sit quietly with your eyes closed for a while and gently bring your focus back to the surroundings.

Autogenic training – stage 1

Close your eyes and repeat the following phrases silently to yourself 3 times each. Think the phrases very slowly and leave a pause before each repetition. Leave a longer pause before you begin the next phrase, so that your mind has time to refocus. If you are going at the right speed, it will take a minimum of 3 minutes, preferably closer to 5 to go through the following phrases. With each phrase let all your focus go to that part of the body.

• My right arm is heavy.
• My left arm is heavy.
• Both my arms are heavy.
• My right leg is heavy.
• My left leg is heavy.
• Both my legs are heavy.
• My arms and legs are heavy.

When you are ready for more, move on to stages 2–6 on pages 122–125.

foods for strengthening the immune system

When you are under par in terms of energy, or are continually getting infections of one type or another, it may be that you have a weak immune system. There are a number of ways to strengthen the immune system. Of these, arguably the single most important is diet. There are certain nutrients your body requires to work efficiently and fight disease.

The World Health Organization has now recognized the importance of the vitamins A, C and E as a means of fighting off disease, from minor infections to several forms of cancer – vitamins that most types of fast food do not provide in sufficient quantity. There are various other vitamins and minerals apart from these that are also essential to good health. Therefore, to maintain a healthy immune system, the advice is to eliminate, or cut down on, highly processed and high-fat foods from your diet, and replace them with fresh natural produce, particularly fruit, vegetables and wholegrains, and a little lean meat and fish.

The diet for this weekend concentrates on these foods. If you can incorporate some of these changes into your normal diet after the Energizing Weekend, you might find it helpful to follow it in a month's time with the Detoxing Weekend and repeat the Energizing Weekend the month after that.

How to eat

The recipes on the following pages are for all of the breakfasts, lunches and suppers this weekend; look through and plan your meals so that you can shop in advance. However, if you consider the fibre and fresh vegetable combination, you can make very quick snacks and suppers.

For breakfast there is a choice of a high-energy drink or muesli; recipes for these can be found on pages 104–105. Try to eat your main meal at lunchtime, as this will give your body time to digest it before bed. A lighter meal, such as a salad, baked potato or soup, is ideal for supper. Whole grains are a good source of nutrients and fibre so choose brown or basmati rice

Drink plenty of fluids – fresh fruit or vegetable juice, bottled or filtered water or herbal teas – so try to drink at least 1.8 litres (3 pints) a day. You should avoid tea and coffee during this weekend.

Make batches of soup in advance and freeze them; defrost when you need a nutritious pick-me-up.

Courgette and ginger soup

SERVES 4

2 tablespoons olive oil

250 g (8 oz) onions, chopped

1.5 kg (3 lb) courgettes, thickly sliced

1 litre (1¾) pints vegetable stock

1 tablespoon grated root ginger

pinch of grated nutmeg

375 g (12 oz) potatoes, sliced

salt and pepper

150 ml (¼ pint) live natural yogurt, to serve

1 Warm the oil in a saucepan over a low heat and cook the onions until soft. Add the courgettes and cook for 5 minutes, stirring.

2 Add the stock, ginger and nutmeg and season with salt and pepper. Bring to the boil, add the potatoes and lower the heat. Simmer, partially covered, for 40–45 minutes.

3 Purée in a blender or food processor, return to the pan and reheat gently. Serve with spoonfuls of yogurt.

Lentil and tomato soup

SERVES 4

425 g (14 oz) can plum tomatoes

2 tablespoons olive oil

1 large onion, chopped

125 g (4 oz) red lentils, rinsed

600 ml (1 pint) vegetable stock

salt and pepper

TO GARNISH

2 tablespoons live natural yogurt

handful of snipped chives

1 Drain the tomatoes, reserving their juice, and chop them roughly.

2 Heat the oil in a saucepan and add the onion. Cook over a low heat until the onion is soft and golden. Stir in the lentils, stock, chopped tomatoes and reserved juice. Bring to the boil, stirring occasionally. Lower the heat, cover and simmer for 15 minutes.

3 Purée in a blender or food processor, return to the pan and season with salt and pepper. Heat through gently and serve garnished with yogurt and chives.

Stuffed peppers

If you are eating alone, you can make the same quantity of filling up to the end of step 2 and freeze the rest.

SERVES 4

300 ml (½ pint) water

½ teaspoon salt

175g (6 oz) brown rice

4 tomatoes, skinned and chopped

1 onion, grated

25 g (1 oz) seedless raisins

75 g (3 oz) Cheddar cheese, grated

2 tablespoons chopped parsley

pinch of ground cinnamon

4 green or red peppers, cored and deseeded, with stem base reserved

5 tablespoons vegetable stock

pepper

1 Bring the water to the boil with the salt, add the rice and cook for 30 minutes, or according to the packet instructions until the rice is tender and all the water has been absorbed.

2 Remove the cooked rice from the heat and gently stir in the onion, tomatoes and raisins. Stir in two-thirds of the grated Cheddar cheese, then the parsley and cinnamon. Season with pepper.

3 If necessary, cut a thin slice off the bottom of each pepper so that it will stand upright. Place the pepper on an ovenproof dish.

4 Divide the rice mixture equally among the peppers, sprinkle with the remaining cheese and cover with the reserved stem bases. Pour the stock around the peppers and cover with foil. Bake in a preheated oven at 200°C (400°F), Gas Mark 6 for 30–40 minutes, until tender.

Tagliatelle with tomato sauce

SERVES 6

2 tablespoons olive oil

2 onions, chopped

2 garlic cloves, crushed

500 g (1 lb) plum tomatoes, skinned and chopped

2 tablespoons tomato purée

125 ml (4 fl oz) vegetable stock

a few ripe olives, stoned and quartered

handful of torn basil leaves

250 g (8 oz) dried tagliatelle

salt and pepper

25 g (1 oz) Parmesan cheese shavings, to garnish (optional)

1 Heat half the olive oil in a large frying pan. Add the onions and garlic and sauté over a low heat until tender, stirring occasionally.

2 Add the tomatoes and tomato purée with the stock, stirring well. Cook over a gentle heat until the mixture is quite thick and reduced. Stir in the olives, basil and season with salt and pepper.

3 Meanwhile, add the tagliatelle to a large pan of boiling salted water. Boil rapidly until the tagliatelle is *al dente*.

4 Drain the tagliatelle, mix in the remaining olive oil and season well with pepper. Put the pasta on a plate, top with the tomato sauce and toss lightly. Serve sprinkled with Parmesan shavings, if liked.

Monkfish salad

SERVES 4

500 g (1 lb) monkfish
fillet, skinned

425 g (14 oz) can
pimentos, drained

5 tablespoons olive oil

1 tablespoon coriander
seeds, crushed

1 onion, sliced

2 garlic cloves, chopped

3 tablespoons capers,
rinsed and drained

pared rind of ½ lemon,
cut into thin strips

125 g (4 oz) Little Gem
lettuce

CORIANDER AND
MINT DRESSING

handful coriander leaves,
torn

handful mint leaves, torn

1 tablespoon balsamic
vinegar

salt and pepper

1 Cut the fish into thin
slices and set aside.
Rinse the pimentos
under cold running
water, drain well and
pat dry with some
kitchen paper. Then, cut
them into strips.

2 Heat the oil in a
frying pan. Add the
coriander seeds and
cook over a low heat
for just a few seconds.
Then toss in the onion
and cook for about
5 minutes, stirring
frequently until soft but
not browned. Add the
garlic and cook for a
minute more.

3 Increase the heat
slightly and add the
fish to the pan. Cook,
stirring gently, for
3–4 minutes, or until the
fish is firm and opaque.

4 Lower the heat, stir
in the pimento, capers
and lemon rind.
Remove the pan from
the heat and allow to
cool for a few minutes.
Remove the monkfish
and set aside.

5 To make the dressing,
add the coriander and
mint to the liquid in the
pan. Add the balsamic
vinegar and season
with salt and pepper to
taste and stir.

6 Serve the fish on a
bed of Little Gem lettuce
leaves, drizzled with the
fresh dressing.

Tuna steaks with avocado

SERVES 2

2 tablespoons olive oil

2 tuna steaks

1 teaspoon chopped
chives, to garnish

mixed salad leaves,
to serve

AVOCADO DRESSING

1 ripe avocado, peeled
and pitted

3 tablespoons live natural
yogurt

1 teaspoon lemon juice

1 Heat the oil in a
frying pan and cook the
tuna steaks gently,
turning frequently, until
they are cooked all the
way through. Remove
from the heat.

2 Meanwhile, make
the dressing. Mash the
avocado in a bowl with
a fork. Mix in the yogurt
and lemon juice.

3 Transfer the tuna to
serving plates and
place a spoonful of the
mixture over each fish.
Garnish with chives
and serve with a salad
of mixed leaves.

Chicken tandoori

SERVES 4

4 chicken breasts, skinned

1 garlic clove, crushed

1 tablespoon tandoori
    powder

300 ml (½ pint) low-fat
    natural yogurt

onion slices, to garnish

mixed salad, to serve

1 Make incisions in the chicken flesh and rub with garlic. Place the chicken in a large shallow bowl. Mix the tandoori powder with the yogurt and toss the chicken in the mixture. Place in the refrigerator to marinate for 3 hours.

2 Heat the grill to moderate. Remove the chicken from the marinade and place it on the grill rack. Grill for about 20 minutes, turning frequently and basting with the reserved marinade.

3 Transfer the chicken to a heated serving dish, garnish with onion slices and serve with a mixed salad.

Spiced fruit

This recipe will keep in the refrigerator for a few days also makes a tasty breakfast. Serve with live, natural yogurt.

SERVES 8

75 g (3 oz) dried apricots

75 g (3 oz) dried peaches

50 g (2 oz) dried figs

50 g (2 oz) sultanas

300 ml (½ pint) apple juice

6 cloves

½ teaspoon grated root
    ginger

1 Chop the apricots and peaches. Remove the stalks from the figs and chop. Put all the fruit into a bowl and cover with the apple juice and spices.

2 Place in the fridge and leave for 3–4 days, serving a bowlful at a time.

Summer pudding

You can keep this in the fridge and have it on consecutive days.

SERVES 4

250 g (8 oz) redcurrants

125 g (4 oz) blackcurrants

125 g (4 oz) raspberries

125 g (4 oz) loganberries

125 g (4 oz) strawberries

125 g (4 oz) cherries or
    blackberries

1 tablespoon clear honey

margarine, for greasing

8 thick slices brown bread,
    crusts removed

1 Place all the fruit in a large saucepan (not aluminium or cast iron) with the honey and cook very gently for 2–3 minutes.

2 Line a lightly greased 1.2 litre (2 pint) pudding basin with three-quarters of the bread, trimming slices to fit so that all the surfaces are completely covered and the base has an extra thick layer.

3 Spoon in all the fruit, reserving 2 tablespoons of the juice in case the bread is not completely coloured by the fruit when the pudding is turned out. Cover with the remaining bread. Lay a plate or lid that will fit inside the rim of the bowl on top and place a 1 kg (2 lb) weight on top. Chill for 10–12 hours.

4 To serve, turn out and cut into wedges.

saturday

8:00 am	**11:30 am**
Autogenic training	Autogenic training
8:30 am	**12:00 am**
Warm-up exercises and	Lunch
stretches	**3:00 pm**
9:30 am	Ayurveda
High-energy drink or	**5:00 pm**
muesli	Autogenic training
10:00 am	**6:00 pm**
Salt scrub	Evening meal
10:30 am	**10:00 pm**
Aromatherapy	Autogenic training

saturday 8:30 am
warm-up exercises and stretches

As soon as you wake up this morning, make yourself a cup of herbal tea. It will rehydrate you and set you up for the day.

The exercises you do each morning after your autogenic training session are based on stretching, which warms up and energizes the body. If you wish, you can leave it at this. But if you are used to regular exercise or fancy getting some fresh air, simply do the warm-up first (see pages 99–101) and then continue with your usual form of exercise or take a brisk walk for at least 20 minutes. Then once you've finished your regular activity, stretch your body afterwards (see pages 102–103). Your muscles will be warmer after physical activity and you will get a better stretch.

Try not to tire yourself out by trying to do more than usual. This weekend is about building more energy than you are expending. If you're not a regular exerciser and want to do some this weekend try brisk walking or rebounding on a mini-trampoline, which gives a tremendous boost to the system, as well as being fun.

Arm stretches

1 Stand tall with a good posture, shoulders relaxed, back straight and navel gently drawn to your spine. Place your feet hip-width apart on the floor.

2 Stretch your left arm straight up to the ceiling. Bend your left knee at the same time, feeling the stretch all the way up your side.

Repeat the stretch on the right side. Do 10 stretches on each side.

Stretch your arms in the same way as before, but this time take your arms out to shoulder level.

Alternate, doing 10 stretches on each side.

Shoulder looseners

1 Stand in the same position as you did for the arm stretches. Slowly roll your shoulders forward towards your chest. Keep your arms relaxed; they will move of their own accord.

2 Lift your shoulders up towards your ears and then move them towards your back, gently squeezing your shoulder blades together. Drop your shoulders back into their natural position. Repeat the exercise 3 more times, then reverse the direction and do another 4 looseners.

Waist twists

1 Stand in the same position as you did for the arm stretches. Fold your arms loosely in front of you so they are about level with your breastbone.

2 Turn to the right from your waist only. Your hips should remain facing squarely to the front. Return to the centre and repeat to the left. Alternate, twisting 10 times to each side.

Side bends

1 Stand as before, with your arms hanging loosely at your sides. Now place your left hand on your hip and raise your right arm.

2 Stretch over to the left, feeling the stretch all the way up the right side of your body.
    Return to the centre and do 8 more stretches on the same side, then repeat on the other side.

Leg swings

1 Stand up straight, feet together at the heels and slightly apart at the toes. Hold on to a chair back with your right hand, if necessary. Lift your left leg and swing it forward.

2 Now swing your leg backwards. Continue swinging your leg backwards and forwards so that your leg is moving in a relaxed way in the hip socket. The hip itself, as well as the upper body, should remain erect and still. You may find it easier to balance if you hold your left arm out just below shoulder level. Do 10 swings, then repeat on your other leg.

This is the end of the warm-up exercises and the point at which you should have some aerobic exercise.

The warm-up prepares your body for exercise. Whatever you do, be active for at least 20 minutes.

Depending on how used you are to exercise, take these stretches as far as feels comfortable. But don't overdo the extent of the stretch or the repetitions.

Back stretch

1 Stand with a straight back, navel drawn lightly to your spine, your shoulders dropped down and feet hip-width apart. Bend forwards from your waist and rest your fingertips on the back of a chair or table. You should just be able to reach it and feel a long stretch in your back. Don't tense your shoulders. Make your back as flat as a table top.

Head rolls

1 Stand up straight, with relaxed shoulders, arms by your sides and your feet hip-width apart. If you can, do this in front of a mirror. Look straight ahead so you are looking into your own eyes.

2 Now, drop your chin on to your chest and feel the stretch up the back of your neck. Hold this position for a moment and try to relax into it.

3 Without tensing or moving your shoulders, roll your head towards your right shoulder. Then take it back to the centre and roll it to the left. Alternate the direction, stretching your neck 4 times on each side.

4 Now lift your head again so you are looking straight ahead. This time, turn your head so that you are looking over your left shoulder. Hold this position for a moment, then turn to the right. Stretch each side 4 times, holding the turned position for a moment each time.

Leg lifts

1 Lie on the floor, with your arms at your sides, legs together. Check you are not tensing any part of your body. Lift your right leg straight up, toes pointing at the ceiling. If you are flexible you can draw it down further, towards your body; use a scarf looped round your ankle, if you like.

Don't try to stretch any further than feels comfortable. Hold the stretch for 1–2 minutes and try to relax into it – your leg will slowly drop down further. Repeat with your left leg.

saturday 8:30 am
cool-down stretches

Diagonal stretch

1 Lie on the floor as in the Leg lifts, but with your arms out at shoulder level. Bend your legs so your feet are flat on the floor and your knees are pointing towards the ceiling.

2 Drop your knees down to the right and, at the same time, turn your head to look to the left. Try to keep your shoulders on the floor. You should feel a strong diagonal stretch across your body. Hold this position for a minute. Return your knees to the centre and drop them to the left, turning your head to the right. Alternate 4 times on each side, holding the stretch each time.

The cat

This is a yoga posture that stretches the spine, thereby promoting strength and flexibility.

1 Kneel on the floor, hands in front, to make a table shape. Your back should be as flat as you can make it and your head in line with your back.

2 Draw your navel to your spine and arch your back upwards, allowing your head to drop down.

Flatten out your back so that it is not curved at all. If you have back problems, do only steps 1 and 2, repeating 4 times. If your back is strong go on step3.

3 Slowly lift your head and push your buttocks up towards the ceiling so that your back forms a concave arch. Look up at the ceiling if you can. Return to a the starting position and repeat the whole sequence 4 more times.

saturday 9:30 am high-energy drink or muesli

This weekend, you can have either muesli for breakfast (see opposite) or a high-energy drink (see below). The drink includes live yogurt, which is good for the digestive system; the fruit and honey give you an immediate boost and go on to release energy throughout the morning.

You can vary the flavour of your shake on a daily basis, simply by changing the fruit. For the sake of sweetness, put in a ripe banana. This makes a delicious drink on its own, but you can then add all other fruit as well. Choose fleshy fruits for a rich, exotic flavour – peaches, apricots, papaya and mango are good for this. For a sharper, fresher taste, try strawberries or raspberries. Very acidic fruits do not really work, but fresh, grated coconut is wonderful.

Try to avoid caffeine this weekend, if you can. If you absolutely must have coffee, have one small cup now, not later in the day. It does give you a boost, but it is a false surge of energy, and eating or drinking your breakfast is a much healthier way to energize. Instead of coffee, have a glass of fresh fruit juice or a herbal tea.

Drink plenty of water throughout the day – at least 1.8 litres (3 pints) – but make sure that you drink only filtered or bottled water.

Yogurt shake
SERVES 1
large glass of live natural yogurt

1 teaspoon honey (up to a tablespoon if you have a very sweet tooth)

fruit, such as banana, peach, mango and strawberries

1 Put all the ingredients in a blender and mix thoroughly.

2 Pour out and drink.

Muesli

This recipe is based on the original version, created by Dr Max Bircher-Benner, a remarkable Swiss physician who made it a staple at his spa. You can add other fruit to the basic recipe: banana is delicious, thinly sliced. All the summer berries give it a fresh flavour, or you can use soaked dried fruit, which makes it a very rich, substantial meal.

2 tablespoons porridge
   oats
2 tablespoons raisins or
   sultanas
4 tablespoons apple or
   pineapple juice
1 apple or pear
1 tablespoon chopped,
   mixed nuts
½ teaspoon ground ginger
1 teaspoon honey
   (optional)
2 tablespoons live natural
   yogurt

1 Soak the oats and raisins or sultanas in the apple or pineapple juice overnight.

2 Next morning, grate the apple or pear and mix into the oats together with the mixed nuts and ginger and, if you have a very sweet tooth, the honey.

3 Pour the yogurt on top of the muesli and serve immediately.

saturday 10:00 am **salt scrub**

This is a gentler version of a treatment found in many European health spas, yet it is still guaranteed to start your day with a boost of energy. A salt body scrub has a number of beneficial effects, all of them stimulating to the system. A salt body scrub:

- clears the pores, sloughs away dead skin cells, so your skin is fresher and smoother
- stimulates the circulation and the elimination of toxins through the lymphatic system
- stimulates cell renewal
- will make your skin tingle and glow with vital energy.

Preparing the salt scrub

There are many exfoliants on the market, yet one of the best is simple salt. You should use rock salt in flakes rather than fine salt (except on the face, see below). You can apply it directly to your body in handfuls, but it is easier to work with if you mix it into a paste with olive or sesame oil. This has the added advantage of nourishing the skin at the same time. You will need a handful of coarse rock salt and 2 tablespoons of olive or sesame oil. If you would like a slightly less functional smell, add 1 drop only of rose or lavender essential oil. Mix all the ingredients together in a bowl and take this with you into the bathroom. Make sure that the bathroom is warm and that you have plenty of warm towels and a towelling robe nearby.

Before you start your body scrub, you should exfoliate your face and neck. For this, you will need to make up a separate mixture, using fine salt, as rock salt will be too coarse for the delicate skin of the face. Use oil even if you have oily skin.

Face scrub

1 Using a face cloth, wet your face and throat with warm water. While it is still wet, massage the scrub mixture into your skin, starting from your throat. Use the first two fingers of each hand to make small circular movements from the base of your throat up to your jaw. Start at the centre and work gradually along the sides.

Apply the scrub mixture over your whole face, except for your eye area. Using the same small circular movements, work along your jaw line from your chin up to your ears.

2 Next, using only the forefinger of each hand, make tiny circles, starting from between your eyebrows, and moving straight up to your hairline; follow your hairline out to your temples. Repeat this from the centre out along the middle of your brow and finally along a line just above your eyebrows out to your temples.

Again, using only your forefingers, exfoliate down the length of your nose and out to the sides, then circle up to the starting point. Repeat this 3 times. Then, starting just below your nose, work out along the edge of your upper lip and then down below your lower lip, and over your whole chin area.

Finally, using the first two fingers of each hand again, exfoliate your cheeks. Start on your cheekbones, working out from your nose towards your ears. Repeat, each time dropping your fingers to a slightly lower starting point until you have exfoliated all your face.

3 Rinse off the salt mixture by splashing lukewarm water all over your face, which should now be soft and glowing.

saturday 10:00 am **salt scrub**

Body scrub

1 Stand under a warm shower for 1–2 minutes and make sure your whole body is wet. Step out from under the water, scoop some of the scrub mixture into your hand and, starting from your feet, massage it well into your skin, using circular movements with your whole hand. Make sure you scrub the soles of your feet, too.

2 Gradually move up your legs, using circular movements all the way. Pay particular attention to your thighs and buttocks as, when the system is sluggish, this is where cellulite is only too likely to appear.

Reach as much of your back as you can and then very gently massage your abdomen and chest.

Finally, scrub your arms and shoulders, as well as your hands themselves.

3 Step back under the shower and massage the scrub into your skin under the water until it has all been washed off. Turn the water temperature down to cold (cool, if you can't face it) and stay under the spray for a further minute, making sure that the water flows over your whole body.

Wrap up in a warm towel and dry vigorously. Put on a warm dressing gown and lie down for 5 minutes. If you feel cold at all, hop back into bed and get under the duvet. You should now feel a tingle all over your body.

saturday 10:30 am **aromatherapy**

Many people think of aromatherapy oils as a cure for problems such as insomnia or anxiety, with an action that is fundamentally calming. But, they can do quite the opposite and pep you up, too.

After your body scrub, make up the Aromatherapy body oil (see opposite), which is designed to give you a lift that will last all day.

Using essential oils

You can fill the room with powerful scents using any of the following methods:
- in a burner, an electric one or one involving a tea-light candle
- in a vaporizer light bulb ring
- directly on a radiator (although this will last for less time and, obviously, works only when the radiator is on).

Uplifting essential oils

One of the best oils is basil, which is particularly stimulating. Others include rosemary, for a more warming, strengthening effect; peppermint, which is both invigorating and soothing, particularly if you are prone to headaches or stomach upsets; and clary sage, which is also an antidepressant. Only use one oil at a time. If you are going out, put 2 drops of one of these oils on a tissue or handkerchief and inhale deeply when you need a pick-me-up when you are flagging.

Caution: Do not use clary sage essential oil if you suffer from high blood pressure.

The best time of day for using all of these oils is the morning. If you use them too late in the day, the effect may be overstimulating and may even cause insomnia. If you have chronic fatigue, caused at least in part by poor sleep, have an aromatherapy bath (see pages 56–57) before you go to bed and do your final autogenic training for the day. A drop or two of lavender oil on a tissue placed on your

pillow will soothe away any tension or anxiety and will help you drift into a blissful sleep.

If you can fall asleep easily but have a problem with waking in the night, try the self-massage on pages 58–59, or put a few more drops of lavender on your pillow – neroli and marjoram are effective, too. Above all, try not to worry about lack of sleep, as the thought may keep you awake. The combination of lavender oil and autogenic training is very successful; just relax and let them take over.

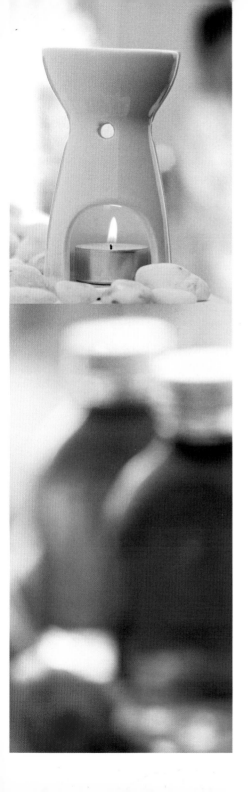

Aromatherapy body oil

- 5 drops of lavender essential oil
- 5 drops of juniper berry oil
- 2 drops of cypress oil

Pour 25 ml (1 fl oz) of carrier oil (grapeseed if you have normal to oily skin; olive or wheatgerm if you have dry or mature skin) into a glass bottle. Add the essential oils listed above to the carrier oil.

This fabulous mixture gives your energy levels a powerful lift for the day, it:
- stimulates the circulation
- purifies the bloodstream
- has a simultaneously calming and uplifting effect.

Massage the scented oil all over your body (except your face) and keep your dressing gown on until all of it has been absorbed.

saturday 3:00 pm **ayurveda**

Ayurveda is traditional Indian medicine, the benefits of which are gradually becoming more widely recognized. One of the most simultaneously energizing and relaxing treatments is *panchakarma*, Ayurvedic massage. There are numerous different forms of *panchakarma* massage, and as more *panchakarma* massage therapists are becoming trained, the massage is becoming more widespread. If you have access to a therapist, book a session as a special weekend treat.

Panchakarma treatments have been found to have remarkable effects on both the mind and the body, which include:
• reducing the risk factors for heart disease and infection
• increasing strength and energy
• improving memory, alertness and sleep patterns.

The basic massage is *abhyanga*, which means 'loving hands'. It usually begins with a head, face and shoulder massage.. This leads on to the body massage. The most surprising features for people used to other forms of massage are that the oil used is hot sesame oil, and that you are massaged by two therapists at once. The effect is hypnotic; tensed muscles seem to become as fluid as the oil pouring over them.

Abhyanga is often followed by *shirodhara*, a treatment which does for your mind what *abhyanga* does for your body. A thin drizzle of sesame oil passes slowly back and forth across your brow, like a pendulum, pausing almost imperceptibly each time it reaches the centre of the temples. *Shirodhara* lasts for 20 minutes and many people compare its effect to transcendence, the meditator's state of bliss. Other treatments include *pinda swedana*, a massage with a sort of rice pudding wrapped in muslin; *urdvartana*, a stimulating, exfoliating massage that increases circulation and promotes weight loss; and *pzzichilli*, in which literally gallons of warm oil are poured continuously over the body while it is gently massaged for around 2 hours.

If you do not have access to a *panchakarma* therapist, there is a certain amount you can try at home. The first thing to aim for is to get the rhythm of your day right. According to ayurveda, every day and every season has a rhythm, and the more you are attuned to it, the healthier and more energized you will feel. For example, an early bedtime is a very important part of the natural daily rhythm. So are rising early and early mealtimes. The main meal of the day should be lunch rather than supper, which should be a lighter meal.

You can try a sesame oil massage at home. If you have a friend who is doing the Energizing Weekend with you, you could take turns to give each other a body massage (see pages 76–78). In this case, however, use sesame oil. Put a small bottle of it in hot water to heat it. The sensation on your skin should be of warmth, so it needs to be allowed to heat for a while.

You can also do a self-massage. Heat the oil in the same way and then, using smooth circular movements, massage it into your whole body. Start with the soles of your feet, then work up your legs, and your body, including as much of your back as you can reach, your arms, your face, scalp and hair. Naturally, your hair will get quite oily, but you can wash it tomorrow morning. The sesame oil is very nourishing for the skin, which will be noticeably softer by tomorrow.

sunday

8:00 am	**11:00 am**
Autogenic training	Autogenic training
8:30 am	**12:00 am**
Warm-up and stretches	Lunch
9:30 am	**3:00 pm**
High-energy drink or	Chi kung
muesli	**5:00 pm**
10:00 am	Autogenic training
Shower with optional	**6:00 pm**
salt scrub	Evening meal
10:30 am	**7:00 pm**
Reflexology	Autogenic training

sunday 10:30 am **reflexology**

Start your day with some autogenic training and the same exercise sessions as yesterday. If you wish, you can repeat yesterday's salt scrub for the body, but not for the face, as this would be too abrasive a treatment to have two days in a row. For breakfast, choose either the yogurt drink or the real muesli, with some juice and herbal tea to rehydrate your body after the long night before.

Take a short break after you eat your breakfast. Read, listen to some music or just relax before your next session, which is a foot massage that encompasses some reflexology techniques.

Reflexology itself requires proper training, but some of the basic movements have been incorporated here. The underlying principle of reflexology is that there are reflex points on the feet that correspond to every organ and part of the body. The theory is that by treating the feet you treat the whole person.

You will find that reflexology:
• has an overall relaxing effect
• stimulates the circulation of blood and lymph.

Many people find that even a simple foot massage makes them so relaxed that they fall asleep. Clearly, this will not happen if you are massaging your own feet but if you do feel tired afterwards, lie down for half an hour before lunch.

Wear loose, comfortable clothes and sit comfortably with your back supported. You will need to find the best position to access each sole of the foot. Some people can sit cross legged with ease; while others prefer to prop the foot they are massaging on the other leg, which is extended in front of them. Use a firm touch throughout.

Caution: Do not practise reflexology if you are pregnant or if you suffer from a heart condition or have varicose veins.

Foot massage

1 Start by relaxing your foot. Hold your foot so that one hand is on the sole and one on the top. Working from your ankle to your toes, massage it with long, firm strokes.

2 Holding your heel in one hand and your toes in the other, circle 5 times clockwise then anticlockwise.

3 Starting with your big toe, stroke the length of each toe in turn and, when you reach the tip, pull gently to stretch it out. Repeat this 3 times.

4 Using your thumb and starting at your big toe, move along the line of pads just below your toes. Press on each one firmly before moving on to the next. Work your way towards your little toe, then change hands and, using your other thumb, work your way back. Repeat twice.

5 Use your thumb to press down gently from the top to the base of your big toe. Repeat on all of your toes. When you reach your little toe, change hands and use the other thumb to go back the other way. Repeat twice.

6 Holding your toes in one hand, use your thumb on the other hand to press along the sole, pressing in a line from the base of your big toe to the centre of your foot, following the line of the metatarsal. Repeat on all your toes, then repeat on the top of your foot following the same line.

7 Starting at your heel, use your thumb to press along the inside edge of your foot all the way up to your big toe. Press firmly and follow the line up over your instep. Then repeat on the outside edge of your foot, from your heel to your little toe.

8 Finally, massage the lower half of your sole, using firm pressure. Rotate your ankle, as before, both clockwise and anticlockwise. Repeat step 1, using long, firm strokes from ankle to toes. Put on a cotton sock and repeat on the other foot.

sunday 3:00 pm **chi kung**

Chi kung is a form of moving meditation and a way of harnessing and releasing the body's own vital energy, or *chi*. It can have an extraordinary beneficial effect on both physical and mental health and it is one of the most energizing forms of exercise. There are many chi kung exercises. Some of them are for specific ailments, but the ones described here increase strength and energy, or *chi*. Given all of this, it is clearly a profound technique and one that cannot be covered in any depth in such a small amount of space.

The best way to learn it is certainly to find a good teacher, go to at least one class a week and practise at home in between. Here, however, are some basic chi kung exercises to serve as an introduction to this remarkable method.

You need to be comfortable and unrestricted for performing chi kung, so dress in loose, cotton clothing and soft shoes, socks or bare feet.

Caution: Do not do these exercises if you are pregnant.

Starting position
Begin in a relaxed standing position. Make sure there is no tension in your spine. Tilt your pelvis slightly forwards to iron out your back and neck, and let your hands hang loosely at your sides. Your neck should follow the line of your spine, so your gaze is straight ahead. Relax your knees.

Lifting the sky

1 From the starting position (see opposite), bring your arms in front of your body, fingertips touching and palms facing the floor.

2 Start to raise your arms out to the sides in a wide circle.

3 When your arms are level with the top of your head, turn the palms to face the ceiling and bring them directly overhead. As far as you can, straighten your arms, with your hands at right angles to your arms, fingertips slightly apart. Hold the stretch for a moment and then lower your arms until your hands are just above your head. Raise and lower in a continuous arc up to 20 times.

Low knee bend

1 Begin in the starting position (see page 116) and open your arms to your sides at shoulder height, palms facing upwards.

2 Breathe in and turn your palms so that they face downwards. Bring your arms up so they stretch straight out in front of you. Start to bend your knees.

3 Breathe out and bend your knees as if you were squatting or sitting on a beach ball.
  Breathe in and return to standing, with your arms still stretched in front of you.

4 Lower your arms to your sides, palms facing backwards. If you feel strong enough, repeat the sequence at least 4 more times.

Embrace the tree

1 Stand in the starting position. Let your knees bend and feel your body's centre of gravity lower, but keep your spine straight.

Slowly raise your arms so they make a wide open circle in front of you, palms facing your chest. Stand in this position for 1 minute (with practice, it would be 5 minutes) and try to relax into it.

Pushing mountains

1 Stand in the starting position (see page 116). Bend your arms at the elbows, with your palms facing forwards, drawing your arms back to the side of your body.

2 Push forwards from the heels of the hands. Draw the arms back again and then repeat up to 20 times.

Plucking stars

1 Stand in the starting position (see page 116). Hold your arms out in front of you, elbows bent, your left arm level with your abdomen, the right at chest level, as if you were holding either side of a beach ball.

2 Lift the left hand upwards, so the two hands pass by each other. When your left hand is level with your face, twist your arm round to allow the palm of your hand to continue to push towards the sky. The right hand should push simultaneously down towards the floor.

3 Push hard enough so that both arms straighten, fingers pointing inwards.

4 Reverse the arms to hold the ball again, this time with your left hand uppermost.

5 Lift the right hand upwards, turning your wrist up. Meanwhile bring your left hand down, to push towards the ground. This is the same position as step 2, but using the opposite arms.

6 Straighten both arms as in step 3. Repeat up to 10 times.

sunday 5:00 pm **autogenic training 2**

You may feel ready to go on to stage 2, or even stage 3, of your autogenic training before the end of the weekend, but there should certainly be no pressure to get further than is absolutely comfortable. The main point of this kind of training is that you relax. If you don't feel completely relaxed with the stage that you are at, don't progress. Wait until you do feel relaxed and then the next stage will give you more benefit.

If you wish, and if you feel ready, you can go on to stage 2 or stage 3 this weekend. However, this is such a useful technique that you will probably want to keep it up, so the next several stages are also outlined below. It is important to emphasize, however, that these should take weeks to achieve. So, go slowly and relax.

Stage 2

When you have practised stage 1 sufficiently and you find yourself going into relaxation very easily, go on to stage 2. Here, you lengthen the session a little by adding one further step. Repeat each phrase slowly, with pauses, as before.

- My right arm is heavy.
- My left arm is heavy.
- Both my arms are heavy.
- My right leg is heavy.
- My left leg is heavy.
- Both my legs are heavy.
- My arms and legs are heavy.
- My neck and shoulders are heavy.

Stage 3

Now a third centre for your focus is added – the breathing. This is not a particularly deep breath but, as you can see from the phrase 'My body breathes me', you become aware of how the breath is affecting your entire body. Again, you first repeat all of the phrases from the previous stage.

- My right arm is heavy.
- My left arm is heavy.
- Both my arms are heavy.
- My right leg is heavy.
- My left leg is heavy.
- Both my legs are heavy.
- My arms and legs are heavy.
- My neck and shoulders are heavy.
- My body breathes me.

sunday 5:00 pm **autogenic training 2**

Stage 4

Do not attempt this stage until you can really feel the focus of the first three. Stage 3, when you add the breathing, usually takes quite a long time to focus on – so give yourself plenty of time. Here, you take the focus to your face; try to feel the sensation of coolness. When you feel ready, go on to the next stage, with the same speed, pauses and repetitions.

- My right arm is heavy.
- My left arm is heavy.
- Both my arms are heavy.
- My right leg is heavy.
- My left leg is heavy.
- Both my legs are heavy.
- My arms and legs are heavy.
- My neck and shoulders are heavy.
- My body breathes me.
- My forehead is cool and relaxed.

Stage 5

Again, don't rush into this stage. Here, you take your focus within to become aware of your heartbeat.

- My right arm is heavy.
- My left arm is heavy.
- Both my arms are heavy.
- My right leg is heavy.
- My left leg is heavy.
- Both my legs are heavy.
- My arms and legs are heavy.
- My neck and shoulders are heavy.
- My body breathes me.
- My forehead is cool and relaxed.
- My heartbeat is calm and regular.

Stage 6

Finally, you take your focus to the mind itself.

- My right arm is heavy.
- My left arm is heavy.
- Both my arms are heavy.
- My right leg is heavy.
- My left leg is heavy.
- Both my legs are heavy.
- My arms and legs are heavy.
- My neck and shoulders are heavy.
- My body breathes me.
- My forehead is cool and relaxed.
- My heartbeat is calm and regular.
- My mind is calm and serene.

There are other elements that can be included and you will certainly be introduced to them if you train with an autogenic training teacher. Here, however, if you have taken it slowly enough, you will have gained enough of the essence of autogenic training for it to be of real and lasting benefit. To continue it in your everyday life, do at least 2 sessions a day and mini-sessions in between if you find yourself having to cope with stressful situations.

Index

Executive Editor Jane McIntosh
Editor Jessica Cowie
Executive Art Editor Jo MacGregor
Designer Ginny Zeal
Senior Production Controller Martin Croshaw

Special Photography: Ian Wallace
Octopus Publishing Group Limited/Jean Cazals
95/Graham Kirk 14, 15, 38, 39, 40, 73, 74/Sandra Lane
front cover top right, 21, 52, 53/Gary Latham 104,
105/William Lingwood 23, 35/David Loftus 20/Diana Miller
54, 94/Peter Myers 13, 55, 72, 75, 96/William Reavell 67
centre right, 67 bottom right/Paul Williams 67 top left